A. Ledda (Ed.)   Vascular Andrology

D1313461

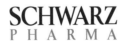

SCHWARZ PHARMA AG · Alfred-Nobel-Straße 10 · 40789 Monheim

Springer

Berlin
Heidelberg
New York
Barcelona
Budapest
Hong Kong
London
Milan
Paris
Santa Clara
Singapore
Tokyo

Andrea Ledda (Ed.)

Vascular Andrology

Erectile Dysfunction, Priapism and Varicocele

With 25 Figures and 12 Tables

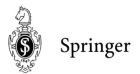 Springer

Dr. Andrea Ledda
Chieti University
Andrology Division
Urology Institute
I-66100 Chieti

Cover illustration
with permission of The Royal Collection
© Her Majesty Queen Elizabeth II

Acknowledgement
This publication has been supported and made possible by a generous grant from
SCHWARZ PHARMA AG, Alfred-Nobel-Str. 10, D-40789 Monheim.
Federal Republic of Germany

ISBN 3-540-59472-8 Springer-Verlag Berlin Heidelberg New York

Die Deutsche Bibliothek – CIP-Einheitsaufnahme
Vascular andology: erectile dysfunction, priapism varicocele; with 12 tables/A. Ledda
(ed.). – Berlin; Heidelberg; New York; Barcelona; Budapest; Hong Kong; London; Milan;
Paris; Santa Clara; Singapore; Tokyo: Springer, 1996
ISBN 3-540-59472-8
NE: Ledda, Andrea [Hrsg.]

SPIN: 10502478   21/3133-5 4 3 2 1 0 – Printed on acid-free paper

Preface

Erectile dysfunction is a complex syndrome associated with and determined by several separate, vascular and nonvascular factors. In recent years the evolution of noninvasive vascular technology for investigating the macro- and microcirculation in vascular disorders has produced a large amount of information and has increased our knowledge of vascular pathophysiology.

In the specific field of vasculogenic erectile dysfunction two major problems have been defined using ultrasound based methods (duplex and color duplex scanning): the first is theoretically caused by decreased arterial inflow and the second by increased venous outflow. Erection is the result of the fine balance and timing between blood inflow and outflow, and these problems often overlap, as both vascular alterations are present in patients with vasculogenic erectile dysfunction.

Recently the role of the microcirculation has been studied using laser Doppler flowmetry and other methods. Preliminary results indicate that microcirculatory alterations may cause vasculogenic impotence even in the presence of a normal (arterial or venous) macrocirculation. In some smokers the presence of diffuse, chronic vasospasm may be a factor in causing erectile dysfunction, which may persist for weeks after smoking has been stopped.

The presence of localized (fibrotic or calcified plaques) or diffuse fibrosis in the corpora cavernosa has recently also been shown using high-resolution B-mode ultrasound. The altered compliance of fibrotic corpora cavernosa may be both an important consequence of an altered perfusion and a significant cause of perfusion alterations.

The role of venous leak has also been investigated, and possibly overstated. It is theoretically and clinically correct to suppose that complex biological and biochemical alterations such as erectile dysfunctions are not caused by a single problem but by a number of factors.

The role of pharmacology and its new interesting developments has also been recently evaluated. The efficacy of new drugs and new formulations or therapeutic solutions can be now quantitatively assessed measuring micro- and macrocirculatory parameters.

In the field of infertility it is now possible to evaluate reliably the presence of asymptomatic varicocele using color duplex. The test is fast and completely noninvasive, and it has been observed that different types of reflux of the pampiniform plexus (e.g., limited proximal reflux, reflux in the whole spermatic cord, diffuse reflux involving the testis) may be associated with different fertility parameters.

A very important recent achievement in this context is presented in this volume, namely, the description of the completely original development of the concept of vascular andrology. As most problems in andrology are related to vascular alterations, the evaluation and – where possible – quantification of these vascular abnormalities has produced a new branch of medical knowledge.

The integrated contributions of important, internationally known clinical research groups has produced a very interesting book, which demonstrates new trends in andrology and underlines the importance of vascular disorders. This volume will be very useful to andrologists, urologists, vascular surgeons, angiologists and to all specialists interested in the diagnostic evaluation of erectile disorders.

GIANNI BELCARO
ANDREA LEDDA

Contents

Part II   Varicocele

Contributors

BELCARO G., M.D.
Microcirculation Laboratory, Cardiovascular Institute,
University of Chieti, Chieti, Italy
Senior Research Fellow, Irvine Laboratory for Cardiovascular
Investigation and Research St.Mary's Hospital Medical
School, Praed Street, London W1, UK

BELGRANO E., M.D.
Professor and Head of Urologic Clinic, University of Trieste,
Cattinara Hospital, Strada di Fiume 447, 34149 Trieste, Italy

BOTTARI A., M.D.
Department of Obstetrics and Gynecology,
SS. Immacolata Hospital, Guardiagrele, Chieti, Italy

CARMIGNANI G., M.D.
Professor and Head of Institute of Urology,
University of Genova, S. Martino Hospital, Genova, Italy

DERIU M., M.D.
Institute of Urology, University of Sassari, Viale Italia 11,
07100 Sassari, Italy

GENTILE V., M.D.
Associated Professor, Institute of Urology,
University La Sapienza of Rome, Rome, Italy

JEREMY J. Y., M.D.
Research Fellow, Department of Chemical Pathology,
Royal Free Hospital and School of Medicine, Pond Street,
London W6, UK

LAURORA G., M.D.
Microcirculation Laboratory, Cardiovascular Institute,
University of Chieti, 66100 Chieti, Italy

LEDDA A., M.D.
Andrology Center, Urologic Clinic, University of Chieti,
SS. Annunziata Hospital, Viale Europe 13, 66100 Chieti, Italy

MENCHINI FABRIS F., M.D.
Professor and Head of Postgraduate School of Andrology,
Institute of Medicine, Policlinico S. Chiara,
University of Pisa, Pisa, Italy

MIKHAILIDIS D., M.D.
Senior Lecturer and Honorary Consultant,
Department of Chemical Pathology,
Royal Free Hospital and School of Medicine,
Pond Street, London W6, UK

SALISCI E., M.D.
Institute of Urology, University of Sassari,
Viale Italia 11, 07100 Sassari, Italy

SIRACUSANO S., M.D.
Institute of Urology, University of Trieste, Cattinara Hospital,
Strada di Fiume 447, 34149 Trieste, Italy

TROMBETTA C., M.D.
Institute of Urology, University of Trieste, Cattinara Hospital,
Strada di Fiume 447, 34149 Trieste, Italy

VALE J.A., M.D.
Consultant Urological Surgeon, St. Mary's Hospital,
Praed Street, London W1, UK

Part I

Erectile Dysfunction

The Prevalence of Vasculogenic Factors in the Aetiology of Erectile Dysfunction

A. Ledda

Introduction

Erectile dysfunction has a multifactorial nature, and in most cases it represents only a symptom of other pathologies. The major causes of physical erectile dysfunction are:

- Diabetes mellitus
- Hypertension
- Smoking
- Vascular disease
- Hypogonadism (and other endocrine disorders)
- High levels of blood cholesterol
- Drugs
- Neurogenic disorders
- Peyronie's disease
- Priapism
- Depression
- Alcohol abuse
- Poor sexual techniques
- Chronic diseases
- Age

Diabetes mellitus, hypertension, smoking, and vascular diseases constitute 80% of all physical causes. Diabetes mellitus affects penile microcirculation and penile nerves, interfering with their normal function and damaging the delicate muscle cells that constitute the erectile tissue. Hypertension and antihypertensive therapies may also damage penile microcirculation. Smoking is the fundamental cause of penile vasospasm.

Vascular diseases and arteriosclerosis may reduce the penile arteriolar blood supply. Even a small reduction in penile blood flow, as well as vasospasm (always present in diabetics and in heavy smokers), can cause erectile dysfunction. Poor arterial supply, vasospasm, fibrosis, and/or small venous anomalies can cause penile veno-occlusive dysfunction and allow excessive drainage of blood from corporal bodies. Vasculogenic factors are certainly the most important of the possible causes of erectile dysfunction.

While many advances have been made in recent years in both the diagnosis and the treatment of erectile dysfunction, a number of aspects remain poorly understood. The likelihood of erectile dysfunction clearly increases with age; however, this is not an inevitable concomitant of aging. Arteriosclerosis also becomes worse with age, but it is possible to slow its progression by altering vascular risk factors. Thus in most cases erectile dysfunction and arteriosclerosis can be said to have the same risk factors, and erectile dysfunction is often but a symptom of an underlying vascular disease. Saenz de Tejada et al. observed in 1988 that "Corporal smooth muscle relaxation results in penile erection through an increase in arterial flow to, and a restriction of venous outflow from the corpora cavernosa." Here we see the three fundamental aspects of penile hemo-dynamic: microcirculation, arteries, and veins.

Even 15 years ago it was still very difficult to perform a complete evaluation of large and small vessels. Today it is possible to quantify all the vascular aspects using noninvasive methods. Microcirculation is easily assessed by laser Doppler flowmetry, and arterial and veinous anomalies can be closely evaluated using echo Doppler or echo color Doppler. Intracavernous injection of vasoactive drugs (e.g., papaverine, phentolamine, prostaglandin) has made an enormous contribution both to the diagnosis and the treatment of erectile dysfunction (National Institutes of Health 1992).

It is our firm belief that treatment of erectile dysfunction must give major priority to vascular risk factors and must only then consider more specific causes. This promises the best prospect of achieving an early and long-lasting solution to erectile dysfunction.

References

Saenz de Tejada I, Goldstein I, Krane RJ (1988) Local control of penile erection. Nerves, smooth muscle and endothelium. Urol Clin North Am 15:9–15

National Institutes of Health (1992) Consensus statement, vol 10, no 4. December 7–9

Vasculogenic Erectile Dysfunction: Diagnosis

A. Ledda, G. Belcaro, and G. Laurora

Introduction

The study of penile hemodynamic parameters has been greatly improved over the past decade by the introduction of intracavernosal injections of vasoactive drugs both in diagnosis and in therapy (Virag 1982). The advent of cavernous pharmacological injections (CPI) has produced a veritable revolution through the contribution which the technique has made in evaluating almost all of the hypotheses on the pathogenesis of vasculogenic erectile dysfunction. Even today great controversy remains concerning the possible correlations between vascular diseases and the inability to achieve a penile erection; although erectile dysfunction may represent a symptom of underlying vasculopathy, the relationship between the two is often influenced by numerous other factors. For example, "performance anxiety" can lead to changes in α-adrenergic tone and congenital alterations in the function of smooth muscle of the sinusoids and other more complex alterations. Nevertheless it is essential to evaluate the vascular risk factors in erectile dysfunction that overlap with those of atherosclerosis; these include cigarette smoking, diabetes, hypertension, and hypercholesterolemia.

Cigarette Smoke

The most widespread vascular risk factor in patients with erectile dysfunction is exposure to cigarette smoking. In many cases cigarette smoke causes peripheral artery disease even before the manifestation of irreversible damage. It can cause vasospasm which is then seen as transient ischemia. There is no such thing as a "safe" cigarette, for even cigarettes extremely low in nicotine can produce a vasospasm phenomena resulting in an unreliable test result. We emphasize the role of cigarette smoking because it is a factor that can be eliminated, and that is involved in an extremely high percentage of cases of male erectile dysfunction (75%–80%), compared with a prevalence of smoking among only 29% of the general population (Ledda et al. 1991, 1992; Virag 1986; Belcaro 1989).

Along with the CPI the first step in the diagnostic protocol is evaluation of the penile circulation by means of a Doppler examination. These tests (echo Doppler and color Doppler), have made an enormous contribution to the diagnostic protocol because they permit the evaluation of the penile arteries, veins, and microcirculation, not only morphologically but also functionally by enabling the measurement of actual blood flow (Figs. 1–3). Today one rarely needs to use angiography, except in patients who have experienced some form of trauma and those patients who are candidates for revascularization (Ledda et al. 1987, 1988, 1989; Lue and Tanagho 1985; Lue et al. 1985).

Physiopathology of Erection

The active role of cavernosal tissue has been evident for more than 100 years. An erection had always been considered a mechanical phenomena and was therefore seen rather simplistically. An erection was regarded as the result of an increase in the arterial blood flow to the corpus cavernosum coinciding with a decrease of the venous return. Normally the arterial blood supply to the corpus cavernosum originates from the internal iliac artery, leading to the internal pudendal artery and terminating with the cavernosal and dorsal arteries (the dorsal terminal branch of the

Fig. 1. Echo color Doppler of penile dorsal artery

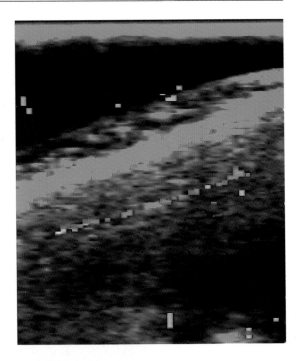

Fig. 2. Echo color Doppler of penile dorsal artery and cavernous artery

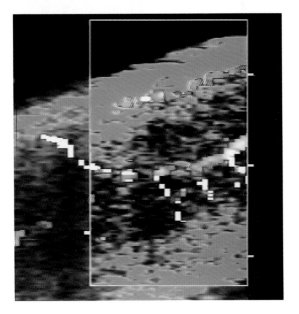

Fig. 3. Echo color Doppler of cavernous artery and fibrosis of cavernous body

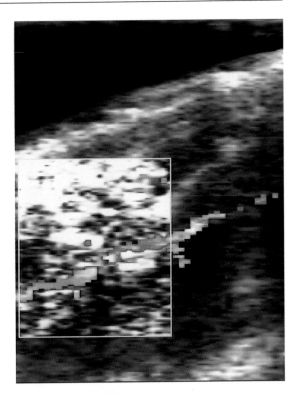

internal pudendal artery). However, there are myriad variations to this from patient to patient.

The venous reflux follows four pathways. The superficial dorsal vein is the principal vessel providing drainage for the glans and the epidermis of the penis, which then empties into the pudendal plexus and/or the saphenous vein. This in turn communicates with the deep dorsal vein, which also drains the glans and the major portion of the corpus cavernosum. Various shunts (communicating veins) exist between the two cavernosal bodies and between these structures and the corpus spongiosum, but they are of minor importance. The deep dorsal vein empties into the periprostatic plexus and the internal pudendal veins. As early as the mid-1980s the crucial role played by the smooth muscle tone of the corpus cavernosum was studied in great detail. The conclusion was reached that alterations in the arteries or veins are of secondary importance with respect to modifications in the smooth muscle tone of the corpus cavernosum (Conti et al. 1988).

With the penis in a flaccid state the smooth muscle of the corpus cavernosum is in an intermediate state between complete relaxation and total contraction. During erection there is a state of relaxation which is translated into an expansion of the sinusoids, which produces a lowering of the peripheral resistance and results in a reduction in the blood flow. A reduction in the venous return is obtained by means of the passive compression of the circumflex veins that are located between the tunica albuginea and the dilated cavernosum tissue. In situations that increase α-adrenergic tone (e.g., cold, anxiety, stress) there is total contraction of the smooth muscles in the cavernosum. An elevated α-adrenergic tone can completely inhibit an erection, even in completely normal healthy subjects (a psychogenic erectile dysfunction can be produced by "performance anxiety"). Studies using the electron microscope have visualized the ultrastructure and the histological morphology and have revealed a degeneration of the smooth muscle of the cavernosum as a primary cause of erectile dysfunction. The smooth muscle tone is regulated by the autonomic nervous system that is derived from the sympathetic and parasympathetic system; the center of the sympathetic system, at the level of the vertebral column, is located in the thoracolumbar region, and the parasympathetic in the sacral region (Conti and Virag 1989).

In addition to the classical neurotransmitters acetylcholine and noradrenaline, other nonadrenergic and noncholinergic neurotransmitters and neuromodulators have been described (e.g., vasoinhibitory peptide, neuropeptide A, calcitonin gene related protein). Recent studies have shown that the neurotransmissions at the corpus cavernosum level are directly related to a vascular mechanism. The cholinergic information as well as the nonadrenergic and noncholinergic appear, at least in part, to be mediated at the endothelial level of the sinusoids which produce the factors that induce both smooth muscle relaxation and the substances that produce their contraction, namely, endothelium- derived relaxing factor and endothelin, which cause contraction. It is thought that nitric oxide or a similar compound mediates the action of endothelium-derived relaxing factor. The endothelial of the sinusoids therefore has an important role in the mechanism of erection. This concept is extremely important, for many common diseases such as diabetes, hypertension, hypercholesterolemia, and atherosclerosis can damage endothelial function even in the very early stages of disease.

Diagnosis

As noted above, until recently there was a lack of diagnostic methods for evaluating patients with erectile dysfunction. However, improvements in old techniques and particularly the introduction of new procedures now permit a more rational and precise therapeutic approach to the patient. The use of invasive methods has all but disappeared.

Figure 4 outlines our diagnostic protocol, which begins with patient history, objective examination, a psychosexual evaluation, and routine blood and hormonal work-ups. The patient history usually orients the physician toward the correct diagnosis. However, one should always continue to the second level of the protocol, CPI with the echo color Doppler. CPI can be performed with various drugs; the most common are papaverine, phentolamine, and prostaglandin E_1. These drugs can be used individually or in combination. In Germany, Austria, and Italy many prefer a cocktail of papaverine (15 mg) and phentolamine (0.5 mg). It is very important to remember that CPI can produce erroneous results if the patient has smoked prior to the examination, or if there are alter-

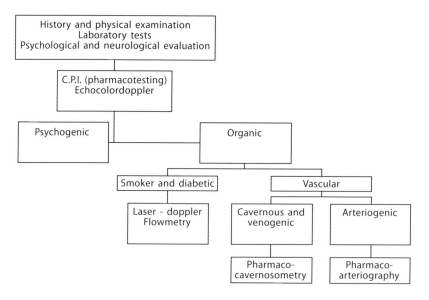

Fig. 4. Diagnostic protocol of vasculogenic erectile dysfunction

ations in the α-adrenergic tone. For this reason CPI examinations must be repeated at least three times, ensuring that the patient is calm and relaxed and has not smoked for at least 7 days prior to the examination. The CPI in association with echo color Doppler is able to show the following: (a) a normal hemodynamic situation in the penis, (b) an arteriogenic origin for the failure to achieve an erection, and (c) the presence of an abnormal pathology of the "occluding vein" mechanism (Ledda et al. 1989; Virag 1982a).

The results of the CPI can be classified using a point system that evaluates the duration and the level of tumescence. Our classification provides for five values: 0, no response to CPI; 1, tumescence; 2, rigidity under 30 min; 3, rigidity between 30 min and 3 h; 4, prolonged erection (over 4 h). Virag (1982b) has defined the arteriogenic form of erectile dysfunction as "erectile attainment deficiency" and the venogenic form as "erectile maintenance deficiency." When the patient begins to react repeatedly to CPI at extremely small doses of medication and with repeated prolonged erections or priapism, the physician should suspect a neurological etiology because this exaggerated reaction is typical of a denerved corpus cavernosum. CPI examinations are indispensable during the course of an echo color Doppler to provide a correct hemodynamic evaluation. Today an evaluation with a duplex probe has become fundamental. In addition to providing information on the morphology and the pathways of the deep dorsal arteries in the corpus cavernosum, it allows the possibility of measuring blood flow in the individual arteries. CPI and the echo color Doppler provide an initial classification of the patient. The peak flow velocities of the cavernosum arteries coinciding with the injection of drugs permits the classification of patients into three groups: less that 20 cm/s, pathological; 20–25 cm/s, borderline (doubtful); greater than 25 cm/s, normal.

The medication used for CPI must be formulated individually. Not all patients respond to CPI using prostaglandin E_1 or the cocktail of papaverine and phentolamine. It is sometimes necessary to repeat the examination several times using various combinations before arriving at the most effective drug and the dose best suited to the patient. We use four combinations for diagnostic CPI: (a) 8 mg papaverine (minitest); (b) 15 mg papaverine + 0.5 mg phentolamine; (c) 15 μg prostaglandin E_1; and (d) 10 mg papaverine + 0.5 mg phentolamine + 10 μg prostaglandin E_1. Normally a very low dose of medication is sufficient to obtain an acceptable dilation of the penile arteries.

An examination that has been the subject of substantial controversy is the penile brachial pressure index (PBI), whose classification is the following: higher that 0.7, normal; corpus cavernosum arteries 0.6–0.7, borderline; lower than 0.6, pathological. Little importance is generally given to this index today, or, rather, to the correlation between the central pressure and the pressure of the cavernosal arteries. However, in our opinion this examination should always be performed. While the PBI may be misleading in the presence of certain pathological conditions, the absolute pressure readings at the level of the penile arteries can always be helpful. The penile pressure reading can be obtained with Doppler or photoplethysmography.

Penile Veno-occlusive Dysfunction

When the patient has a repeatedly negative response to the various types of CPI, a vascular origin of the erectile dysfunction should be suspected. In the presence of normal arterial input and an apparently intact microcirculation one should suspect a venous escape defined as an occluding vein dysfunction of the corpus cavernosum. Usually a dysfunction of this nature is studied by means of pharmaco-cavernosometry, which, however, is an invasive examination and is very uncomfortable for the patient. In recent years there have been increased efforts to diagnose this form of erectile deficit more rapidly through the use of noninvasive examinations. Numerous researchers have directed their attention to the values of end-diastolic velocity, peak systolic velocity, and resistance index. The reason for this is that there is an alteration in these hemodynamic parameters in all patients affected by a dysfunction of the occluding vein mechanism in the corpus cavernosum. The velocity of the blood flow is decisive, while the diameter of the corpus cavernosum arteries is usually not measured due to the small dimensions of these vessels. The relationships among these variables are defined as: resistance index=peak systolic velocity minus end-diastolic velocity divided by peak systolic velociy. The latest generation of echo color Doppler can furnish this information and calculate these values. The person performing the test needs only to identify the vessels to be examined and to position the sampling volume of these vessels. It is more important than in other forms of erection dysfunction that a careful evaluation be made of the possible correlation between the clinical picture and the results of ultrasonography. Lue (Lue et al. 1985) has observed that one examination is not sufficient to arrive at a diagnosis since all of these techniques are associated with a high rate of false-positive and false-negative results. The reliability of the evaluation is based upon the sum of all the available data and upon a critical interpretation of the numeric values and results of the various examinations. The controversy between the supporters of pharmaco-cavernosometry and supporters of penile echo color Doppler is very animated. In our experience, however, these techniques should be used to complement one another. Technically the problem is to create a situation that will render the evaluation more reliable (Tenaglia et al. 1989).

When the penis is in a flaccid state there is no measurable diastolic flow, and the index of resistance is less than 1. Upon relaxation of the sinusoids and the onset of an erection the diastolic flow increases and the resistance index then decreases. Once a state of a complete erection has been reached, the diastolic flow approaches a value of 0, and the resistance index again increases, approaching or returning to a value of 1. If venous occlusion is not complete, the resistance index is less than 1. Resistance during the flaccid state is determined by the sinusoids, while resistance during an erection is determined by the occlusion of the venous plexus and particularly of the circumflex veins. It is evident that the mechanism of occlusion of the circumflex veins can in turn be compromised by an inadequate dilatation of the sinusoids. The causes of this phenomenon include all the factors that can lead to vasospasms and alterations of the α-adrenergic tone. The smooth muscle can be susceptible to neurological diseases, cigarette smoke, psychological inhibition, medication, and congenital diseases of the smooth muscle.

Under some conditions, wich can occur in patients affected by induratio penis plastica or fibrosis or in those who have a transient or chronic contraction in the smooth muscles of the corpus cavernosum, the intracavernosum pressure is not able to increase sufficiently to compress the circumflex veins and to maintain the erection. Therefore, it is necessary to distinguish between patients in whom there is a pathology only in the venous "output" and those in whom there coexist sinusoidal alterations and/or alterations of the arterial input. Patients with an arterial occluding vein dysfunction who also have a systolic peak less than 25 cm/s during echo Doppler are definitely poor candidates for venous surgery because it would be useless to reduce the venous return artificially in the presence of concomitant low arterial flow.

Conclusion

The differential diagnosis for erectile dysfunction has been greatly simplified and at the same time has become more reliable with the introduction of CPI and echo Doppler. Patients with normal hemodynamic parameters can be examined in less than 30 min by means of an inexpensive, noninvasive technique without having to resort to complex protocols as was the case until only a few years ago. Color has greatly simplified the examination, enabling even the patient to comprehend the results. The patient is reassured, and in the case of a normal hemodynamic situation he can be started immediately on psychosexual therapy or treatment with vasodilators. The simplicity and assurance of a proper diagnosis undoubtedly reflect on the therapeutic indications, which today are also more accurate.

It should not be forgotten that erectile dysfunction is often the symptom of an underlying vascular pathology, and it is always recommended that the patient undergo a general vascular study, including an ultrasonic arterial biopsy (Fig. 1, p. 61). Ultrasound biopsy is an effective screening method for detecting early, subclinical arteriosclerotic lesions. Carotid and femoral artery wall lesions are important markers of generalized cardiovascular disease. The evaluation of four arterial sites (both carotid and femoral arteries) gives a clue as to the status of the whole cardiovascular system. In 27.9% of patients, the femoral lesions are present earlier or in a more advanced stage than carotid lesions. Different age groups have a different ultrasound biopsy class distributions and scores due to the age-related progression of the disease. Early arterial lesions and small plaques are important indicators of silent coronary ischemia and cardiovascular events. The method also has an impact on patients' compliance. We believe that ultrasound biopsy should be performed on all the patients with suspected vasculogenic erectile dysfunction.

References

Belcaro G (1989) Flussimetria laser-doppler e microcircolazione. Minerva Medica, Turin

Castronuovo J Jr, Pabst TS, Flamigan DP, Foster LS (1987) Non invasive determination of skin perfusion pressure using laser doppler. J Cardiovasc Surg 28:253-257

Conti G, Virag R (1989) Human penile erection and organic impotence: normal histology and histopathology. Urol Intern 44:303-308

Conti G, Virag R, Von Niederhausen W (1988) The morphological basis for the polster theory of penile vascular regulation. Acta Anat 133:209-212

Ledda A, Belcaro G, Laurora G, Gabini M (1987) Valutazione dell'impotenza erettile con tests non-invasivi. Fifth Congress of the Italian National Society on Andrology, Bologna, pp 777-779

Ledda A, Belcaro G, Rossetti R, Seccia M et al (1988) Methods of quantitative evaluation of flow in andrology. XXVI Congress of the International College of Surgeons, Milan, 3-9 July, 1988. Monduzzi, Milan, p 341

Ledda A, Belcaro G, Martegiani C et al. (1989) Il duplex scanning in andrologia. S.U.I.C.M.I, Sorrento 1988. Acta Urol Italica

Ledda A, Tenaglia R, Belcaro G (1991) Laser doppler in impotent smokers. Arteres Veines 10:179-180

Ledda A, Laurora G, Belcaro G (1992) The evaluation of penile perfusion pressures by laser-doppler flowmetry. Fifth World Congress on Impotence, Milan 14-17 September 1992. Int J Impotence Res 4 [Suppl 2]:89

Ledda A, Seccia M, Martegiani C et al (1989) 18 mesi di esperienza con le farmacoprotesi peniene. 61st Congress S.I.U., Cagliari 1988. Acta Urol Italica 4 [Suppl 1]

Lue TF, Tanagho EM (1985) Functional evaluation of erectile impotence. Acta Urol 16:244

Lue TF, Hricak H et al (1985) Vasculogenic impotence evaluated by high-resolution ultrasonography and pulsed doppler spectrum analysis. Radiology 155:777

Tenaglia R, Ledda A, Martegiani C (1989) Impotenza venosa: un nuovo approccio diagnostico non invasivo. XXXVIII Conference of the Society of Urologists in Northern Italy. Trento, 13 June 1989

Virag R (1986) Impuissance et tabac. Tabac 64:6-16

Virag R (1982a) Intracavernous injection of papaverine for erectile failure. Lancet 2:938

Virag R (1982b) Arterial and venous hemodynamics in male impotence. In: Bennet (ed) Management of male impotence. pp 108-126

Prostaglandins and the Aetiology and Treatment of Erectile Dysfunction

J. Y. Jeremy and D. P. Mikhailidis

Introduction

Both animal and human penile tissue synthesize prostaglandins (PGs). Furthermore, intracavernous injection of certain PGs elicits erection in men with erectile dysfunction (ED; Godschalk et al. 1994). It is also well established that PGs are involved in the pathophysiology of atherosclerosis. Since atherosclerosis is a major cause of ED (Virag et al. 1985), it has been suggested that disruption of PG synthesis in penile tissues and related vasculature may play a role in the pathogenesis of ED (Jeremy and Mikhailidis 1990). The present chapter therefore focuses on the role of PGs in normal penile erection as well as on the pathophysiology and treatment of ED with PGs and related drugs. Several recent reviews on these areas are of interest (Juenemann and Alken 1989; Jeremy and Mikhailidis 1990; Linet 1993; Miller and Morgan 1994).

Biosynthesis and Properties of Prostaglandins in Blood Vessels

Since this chapter focuses on vasculogenic impotence, and a great deal is known of the control of PG synthesis in blood vessels and their role in vascular disease, this topic is included as a primer to the discussion of PGs in the penis.

Blood vessels synthesize a range of PGs, principally (listed in general quantitative rank order): PGI_2, PGE_2, PGD_2, $PGF_{2\alpha}$ and thromboxane A_2 (TXA_2; Jeremy et al. 1988). Although the constrictor or dilator activity of individual PGs varies between species and vessel types, in most vessels PGI$_2$, PGE$_2$ and PGD$_2$ are vasodilators and PGF$_{2\alpha}$ and TXA$_2$ are vasoconstrictors. PGE$_1$ has a biphasic effect, with vasodilation at high doses. Inhibitors of PG synthesis, such as aspirin and indomethacin, have been shown to increase basal vascular tone and to attenuate responses to dilator (antihypertensive) agents (Hadhazy et al. 1988). The latter observation suggests that the principal role of endogenous vascular PGs is that of vasodilation.

It is also notable that PGs, in particular PGI$_2$ and PGE$_{2\alpha}$, play other roles in atherogenesis. For example, PGI$_2$ inhibits platelet and leukocyte adhesion, reduces cholesterol accumulation in vascular cells and inhibits proliferation of vascular smooth muscle cells (Jeremy 1994). Since all these processes are key pathological events in atherogenesis, PGs are likely to influence ED indirectly through the roles that they play in atheromatous disease of penile tissue and associated blood vessels.

Prostaglandins and Normal Penile Function

That PGs may play a role in erection and detumescence was first indicated by Klinge and Sjostrand (1977) who found that PGF$_2$ induces contraction of isolated corpus cavernosum as well as the penile artery and retractor penis muscle of bulls. Subsequently it was found that the animal and human corpus cavernosum produces a range of PGs including PGF$_{2\alpha}$, PGE$_2$, PGI$_2$ and TXA$_2$ (Roy et al. 1984; Jeremy et al. 1986a,b; Saenz de Tajeda 1988). It was also demonstrated that muscarinic (but not adrenergic) stimulation of both animal and human penile tissue results in the release of PGI$_2$ (Jeremy et al. 1986a,b). Since PGI$_2$ is a vasodilator, at least in vascular tissues other than the penis, it has been proposed that the release of PGI$_2$ may be involved in the vasodilatory phenomenon associated with erection (a partially cholinergic process). As a potent inhibitor of platelet adhesion and aggregation, acute release of PGI$_2$ may also protect the penis from thrombosis during engorgement of the penis.

In an elegant study on isolated human penile tissue, Hedlund and Andersson (1985) established that PGs elicit different effects on human corpus cavernosum, corpus spongiosum and corpus cavernosal artery.

$PGF_{2\alpha}$, PGI_2 and TXA_2 analogues contract corpus cavernosum and corpus spongiosum whereas PGE_1 and PGE_2 (but not PGI_2) relaxes the corpus cavernosum and spongiosum (when precontracted with noradrenaline or $PGF_{2\alpha}$). Thus, based on these data it would appear that PGI_2 is unlikely to be a major relaxant mediator during erection. This is borne out by experiments in which intracavernosal injection of PGI_2 in monkeys in vivo at bolus doses of 100–200 μg did not increase the arterial blood flow, and indeed the concomitant smooth muscle contraction produced a large reduction in cavernosal compliance (Bosch et al. 1989). This is in contrast to the increased cavernosal arterial blood flow and cavernosal smooth muscle relaxation elicited by intrapenile injection of PGE_1 in monkeys and rats (Bosch et al. 1989; Chen et al. 1992). This disparity between the effects of PGI_2 and PGE_1 is surprising since these two PGs possess very similar properties in other tissues (e.g. inhibition of platelet function, relaxation of blood vessels; Willersen et al. 1994). However, in the penis this could be due to different populations of receptors. Indeed, recent evidence suggests that endogenous PGE_1 receptors in the penis play an important role in erection and ED (Aboseif et al. 1993). PGE_1 has also been shown to inhibit noradrenaline release from penile adrenergic nerves (Molderings et al. 1989). We have recently shown that PGE_1 stimulates the synthesis of cyclic adenosine-3′,5′-monophosphate (cAMP) in the rat penis and proposed this event to be the principal mechanism that mediates the erectogenic effect of PGE_1 (Miller et al. 1994).

Apart from prostanoids, it has become increasingly apparent that other endogenous non-cholinergic, non-adrenergic vasoactive substances play a role in the normal erection and the pathophysiology of ED. These include nitric oxide (NO), vasoactive intestinal polypetide, purinergic agonists (e.g. adenosine), endothelin and neuropeptide Y (Miller and Morgan 1994). Detailed discussion of these factors, however, is beyond the scope of the present article, but nevertheless warrant consideration when investigating the pathophysiology of vasculogenic ED.

Pathogenesis of Impotence: Possible Role of PGs

Virag et al. (1985), in an extensive 'epidemiological' study, highlighted the role of arterial lesions (atheroma) as a cause of ED. This seminal paper has led to the distinct category of 'vasculogenic' in classifying and diagnosing cases of ED. Epidemiologically, diabetes mellitus (DM), cigarette smoking, hyperlipidaemia and hypertension are major risk factors for both ED and atherosclerosis and where present together exert a cumulative effect on the likelihood of developing ED (Ledda et al. 1991; Miller and Morgan 1994; Mikhailidis and Jeremy 1994; Jeremy 1994).

DM exerts powerful deletrious effects on the neural and vascular elements of erection and as such is a very strong risk factor for ED (50% of diabetics over 50 years have ED; McCulloch 1980). DM is also classically associated with disruption of PG synthesis (Mikhailidis et al. 1988; Hendra and Betteridge 1988; Horrobin 1988). Streptozotocin-induced DM in the rat results in a marked inhibition of PGI_2 synthesis by both penile and vascular tissues (Jeremy et al. 1985). These effects relate to duration rather than severity, thus mirroring the human situation (Jeremy et al. 1986c). Furthermore, the reduced PGI_2 synthesis is reversed to normal by administration of insulin (Jeremy et al. 1985). Aboseif et al. (1993) have also recently reported a reduction in PGE_1 receptors in penile tissues from diabetic men. In this context, we recently found that PGE_1-stimulated cAMP synthesis by both the penis and aorta of the diabetic rat is markedly enhanced in DM (Miller et al. 1994). It was reasoned that this effect is due to an upregulation of adenylate cyclase activity, and the enhanced production of cAMP may be an adaptive event aimed at countering the deleterious effects of DM on pro-erectile mechanisms (e.g. attenuation of dilator receptor activity at the plasma membrane level). We also found that the activity of the enzyme cAMP phosphodiesterase (PDE) is diminished in the penis of the diabetic rat (Miller et al. 1995). Since PDE hydrolyses cAMP to inactive AMP, diminished activity of this enzyme would also effectively enhance cAMP levels. Furthermore, we found that 5'-nucleotidase activity (generating adenosine from AMP) is enhanced in the penis of diabetic rats (Khan et al. 1994). Since adenosine is a potent vasodilator, the upregulation of this enzyme's activity in DM may constitute an additional adaptive mechanism.

Cigarette smoke extracts have been shown to inhibit penile PGI_2 synthesis (Jeremy et al. 1986c). Moreover, this cigarette smoke-induced inhibition is additive to the inhibition of this prostanoid in DM (Jeremy et al. 1986d), which mimics the situation in patients. It is notable that cigarette smoking adversely affects penile arterial blood flow, causing acute vasoconstriction (Hirschowitz 1992). These effects may be compounded by a lowered arterial oxygen tension which affects NO synthase (Kim et al. 1993), and penile receptor-mediated responses (Broderick et al 1994).

It has long been recognized that hyperlipidaemia is a major risk factor for the development of atherosclerosis and ED (Virag et al. 1985). However, it has only recently been demonstrated that hypercholesterolaemia results in penile smooth muscle and endothelial dysfunction in an animal model of penile atheroma (Kim et al. 1994). In turn, hyperlipidaemia is associated with disruption of both PG and NO synthesis at the vascular endothelial level (Jeremy 1994). In the context of a recent report of favourable changes in vessel reactivity following administration of lipid-lowering drugs (Leung et al. 1993), it is reasonable to speculate that hyperlipidaemia may contribute to ED via an attenuation of the vasodilator action of PGs at the endothelial level. This hypothesis also raises obvious therapeutic implications.

Therapeutic Use of PGs and Related Drugs in Erectile Dysfunction

Intracavernosal injection of PGE_1 in the treatment of ED was first described by Stackl et al. (1988) and Ishii et al. (1989). Juenemann and Alken (1989) concluded that papaverine may cause unwanted prolonged erection in up to 9.5% of patients, while PGE_1 is associated with a considerably lower rate of 2.4%. PGE_1 is also effective in a proportion of cases which do not respond to papaverine and has an overall response rate of 70%–80% (Juenemann and Alken 1989; Linet 1993). A major drawback of PGE_1 is the significant incidence of local pain after cavernosal injection, in as many as 40% of patients (Linet 1993). Nevertheless, PGE_1 is undoubtedly safer than other pharmacological agents since it is rapidly degraded to inactive metabolites by endogenous enzymes. Because of this property PGE$_1$ also exerts minimal systemic side effects following intra-penile injection. It is also of interest that in a recent comparison between linsidomine (a NO donor) and PGE$_1$, linsidomine elicited only modest erections compared to PGE$_1$ (Porst 1993).

It may also be possible to enhance endogenous penile PGE$_1$ synthesis by dietary supplementation with the naturally occurring precursor of this prostanoid, γ-linolenic acid. In this context, γ-linolenic acid (as a principal component of evening primrose oil) has been shown to enhance the synthesis of PGE$_1$ in other tissues (Horrobin and Manku 1990), and such may be the case in the penis. Evening primrose oil has also been shown to improve nerve function in patients with diabetic neuropathy and to be protective against peripheral nerve dysfunction in animal models of DM (Cameron et al. 1993). Given this dual property of γ-linolenic acid, long-term dietary supplementation with evening primrose oil may prove useful in ameliorating ED, particularly in DM where this condition is prevalent. We are unaware of any rigorous studies of this type of supplementation in ED. However, given its success in the treatment of other vascular diseases, investigations into the possible beneficial effect of evening primrose oil warrants consideration.

As described above, PGE$_1$ is a potent elevator of intracellular levels of cAMP in penile tissue (Miller et al. 1994). Thus, another class of drugs which may prove useful in the treatment of ED are the PDE inhibitors (e.g. milrinone, isobutylmethylxanthine; Jeremy et al. 1993). PDEs, rapidly hydrolyse cAMP to the inactive metabolite AMP. PDE inhibitors thus act as vasodilators by effectively elevating tissue levels of cAMP. Indeed, we have recently found that papaverine itself is an inhibitor of cAMP PDE, albeit at high concentrations (Jeremy et al., unpublished observations), which may explain its efficacy as an erectogen. The pharmaceutical industry is also developing novel and potent cyclic GMP PDE inhibitors. Since the action of NO is ultimately mediated by elevation in cyclic GMP, cGMP PDE inhibitors may prove useful in the treatment of ED. It is also possible that orally administered PDE inhibitors could enhance the efficacy of erectogens which are injected intracavernosally, and whose actions are mediated by increased tissue levels of cyclic nucleotides.

Finally, as was described earlier, several clinical conditions predispose to the development of ED (DM, hyperlipidaemia, hypertension, tobacco addiction). Such patients could therefore be monitored for early signs of ED and their risk factors controlled, for example, by administration of lipid-lowering drugs and antihypertensive drugs (Miller et al. 1993). High-risk patients should also be counselled vis-à-vis life-style, in particular, diet and the smoking habit. Such an approach may also confer an overall survival benefit in such patients.

References

Aboseif S, Riemer RK, Stackl W, et al (1993) Quantification of PGE$_1$ receptors in cavernous tissue of men, monkeys and dogs. Urol Int 50:48–152

Bosch RJLH, Benard F, Aboseif SR (1989) Changes in penile hemodynamics after intra cavernous injection of PGEl and prostaglandin I2 in pig-tailed monkeys. Int J Impotence Res 1:211–221

Broderick GA, Gordon D, Hypolite L, Levin RM (1994) Anoxia and corporal smooth muscle dysfunction: a model for ischaemic priapism. J Urol 151:259-262

Cameron NE, Cotter MA, Dines KC et al (1993) The effects of evening primrose oil on nerve function and capillarization in streptozotocin diabetic models modulation by the cyclooxygenase inhibitor, flurbiprofen. Br J Pharmacol 109:972–979

Chen KK, Chan KY, Chang LS, et al (1992) Intracavernous pressure as an experimental index in a rat model for the evaluation of penile erection. J Urol 147:1124–1128

Godschalk MF, Chen Z, Katz PG, Mulligan T (1994) Treatment of erectile failure with prostaglandin El: a double blind placebo-controlled, dose response study. J Urol 151:1530–1536

Hadhazy P, Malomvolgyi B, Magyar K (1988) Endogenous prostanoids and arterial contractility. Prostaglandins Leukot Essent Fatty Acids 32:175–187

Hedlund H, Andersson K (1985) Contraction and relaxation induced by some prostanoids in isolated human penile erectile tissue and cavernous artery. J Urol 134:1245–1250

Hendra T, Betteridge DJ (1988) Platelet function, platelet prostanoids and vascular prostacyclin synthesis in diabetes mellitus. Prostaglandins Leukot Essent Fatty Acids 35:197–212

Hirschkowitz M, Karacan I, Howell W, et al (1992) Nocturnal penile tumescence in cigarette smokers with erectile dysfunction. Urol 39:l0l-107

Horrobin DF (1988) The roles of fatty acids in the development of diabetic neuropathy and other complications of diabetes mellitus. Prostaglandins Leukot Essent Fatty Acids 31:181–197

Horrobin DF, Manku MS (1990) Clinical biochemistry of essential fatty acids. In: Horrobin DF (ed) Omega-6 fatty acids: pathophysiology and roles in clinical medicine. Liss, New York, pp 21–54

Ishii N, Watanabe H, Irisawa C, et al (1989) Intracavernous injection of PGE1 for the treatment of erectile impotence. J Urol 141:323–325

Jeremy JY (1994) Smoking and vascular defence mechanisms. J Smoking Related Disorders 5 [Suppl 1]: 49–54

Jeremy JY, Mikhailidis DP (1990) Prostaglandins and the penis: possible role in impotence. Sex Marital Ther 5:155–165

Jeremy JY, Mikhailidis DP, Thompson CS, Dandona P (1985) Experimental diabetes mellitus inhibits prostacyclin synthesis by the rat penis: pathological implications. Diabetologia 28:365–368

Jeremy JY, Morgan RJ, Mikhailidis DP, Dandona P (1986a) Prostacyclin synthesis by the corpora cavernosa of the human penis: evidence for muscarinic control and pathological implications. Prostaglandins Leukot Essent Fatty Acids 23:211–216

Jeremy JY, Morgan RJ, Mikhailidis DP, Dandona P (1986b) Muscarinic stimulation of prostacyclin synthesis by the rat penis. Eur J Pharmacol 123:67–71

Jeremy JY, Thompson CS, Barradas MA, Mikhailidis DP, Dandona P (1986c) Duration but not severity determines effects on prostacyclin synthesis in the rat aorta, penis and bladder. Prog Lipid Res 25:505–507

Jeremy JY, Thompson CS, Mikhailidis DP, Dandona P (1986d) The effect of cigarette smoke and diabetes mellitus on muscarinic stimulation of prostacyclin synthesis by the rat penis. Diabetes Res 3:467–469

Jeremy JY, Mikhailidis DP, Dandona P (1988) Excitatory receptor-linked prostanoid synthesis in mammalian smooth muscle: the role of calcium, protein kinase C and G proteins. Prostaglandins Leukot Essential Fatty Acids 34:215-228

Jeremy JY, Gill J, Mikhailidis DP (1993) Effect of milrinone on human platelet cAMP phosphodiesterase, iloprost cAMP, thromboxane A2 synthesis and calcium uptake. Eur J Pharmacol 245:67–73

Juenemann K, Alken P (1989) Pharmacology of erectile dysfunction: a review. Int J Impotence Res 1:71–93

Khan N, Miller M, Thompson CS, Mikhailidis DP, Morgan RJ, Jeremy JY (1995) 5' nucleotidase activity in the aorta and penis of the diabetic rat. J Mol Cardiol (in press)

Kim N, Vardi Y, Padma-Nathan H, et al (1993) Oxygen tension regulates the nitric oxide pathway. J Clin Invest 91:437–442

Kim J, Klyachkin ML, Svendsen E, et al (1994) Experimental hypercholesterolaemia in rabbits induces cavernosal atherosclerosis with endothelial and smooth muscle cell dysfunction. J Urol 151:198–205

Klinge E, Sjostrand NO (1977) Comparative study of some isolated smooth muscle effectors of penile erection. Acta Physiol Scand 100:354–367

Ledda A, Tenaglia R, Belcaro G (1991) Laser-Doppler flowmetry in impotent smokers. Arteres et Veines 10: 179–180

Leung W, Lau C, Wong C (1993) Beneficial effect of cholesterol-lowering therapy on coronary endothelium-dependent relaxation in hypercholesterolaemic patients. Lancet 341:1496–1500

Linet OI (1993) Prostaglandins in erectile dysfunction. In: Vane JR and O'Grady J (eds) Therapeutic applications of prostaglandins. Arnold, Boston, pp 105–121

McCulloch DK, Campbell IW, Wu FC (1980) The prevalence of diabetic impotence. Diabetologia 18:279–283

Mikhailidis DP, Jeremy JY (1994) Smoking and Impotence. Int Angiol 12:297–298

Mikhailidis DP, Jeremy JY, Dandona P (1988) The role of prostaglandins, leukotrienes and essential fatty acids in the pathogenesis of the complications associated with diabetes mellitus. Prostaglandins Leukot Essent Fatty Acids 33:205–206

Miller MAW, Morgan RJ (1994) Eicosanoids, erections and erectile dysfunction. Prostaglandins Leukot Essent Fatty Acids 51:1–9

Miller MAW, Morgan RJ, Thompson CS, Mikhailidis DP, Jeremy JY (1994) Adenylate and guanylate cyclase activity in the penis and aorta of the diabetic rat: an in vitro study. Br J Urol 74:106–111

Miller M, Morgan RJ, Thompson CS, Mikhailidis DP, Jeremy JY (1995) Alterations of phosphodiesterase activity in the penis and aortae of diabetic rats (abstract). Int J Impotence Res (in press)

Miller MAW, Thompson CS, Jeremy JY (1993) Managing impotence in diabetes-no need for a service. Br Med J 307:738

Molderings GJ, Gothert M, Van Ahlen H, Porst H (1989) Noradrenaline release in human corpus cavernosum and in modulation via presynaptic alpha adrenoceptors. Fundam Clin Pharmacol 102:261–267

Porst H (1993) PGE1 and nitric oxide donor linsidomine for erectile failure: a diagnostic comparative study of 40 patients. J Urol 149:1280–1283

Roy AC, Tan SM, Kottegoda SR, Ratnam SS (1984) Ability of the human corpora cavernosa muscle to generate prostaglandins and thromboxanes in vitro. IRCS J Med Sci 12:608–609

Saenz de Tajeda I, Goldstein I, Krane RJ (1988) Local control of penile erection. Nerves, smooth muscle and endothelium. Urol Clin North Am 15:9–15

Stackl W, Hasun R, Marberger M (1988) Intracavernous injection of PGE1 in impotent men. J Urol 140:66–68

Virag R, Bouilly P, Frydman D (1985) Is impotence an arterial disorder? A study of arterial risk factors in 440 impotent men. Lancet I: 181–184

Willersen JT, Sheng-Kun Y, McNatt J, et al (1994) Liposome-bound prostaglandin E1 often prevents cyclic flow variations in stenosed and endothelium-injured canine coronary arteries. Circulation 89:1786–1791

Evaluation of Penile Microcirculation

A. Ledda and G. Belcaro

Introduction

Penile arterial and venous circulation has been widely investigated, using various techniques including echo Doppler, echo color Doppler, photoplethysmography, angiodynography, cavernosometry, arteriography, and isotope wash-out techniques. Penile microcirculation, on the other hand, has been less extensively investigated both in physiological and in pathological conditions. The introduction of laser Doppler flowmetry (LDF) in the past decade has provided a useful means to evaluate microcirculation in normal and pathological conditions. LDF is also used to evaluate the effects of vasoactive drugs and the superficial skin microcirculation in patients with vasculogenic erectile dysfunction. The technique is extremely easy to handle and has become very popular; however, the interpretation of results is sometimes rather critical.

LDF allows movements of particles of a certain, minimal mass to be measured (Fagrell 1994). In living tissue all particles including blood cells that move can be recorded. It is extremely important to distinguish between the measurement of blood velocities in larger, discrete vessels and that of blood perfusion at a microvascular level. Both measurements are possible using LDF, but all presently available LDF devices are designed to measure only microvascular blood perfusion and pressure. A very important advantage of LDF over other methods of monitoring circulation is that it directly measures the delivery of blood to the tissue (Borgos 1994). In many pathological conditions this may be of more value to clinicians. The LDF evaluation of vasculogenic erectile dysfunction provides better understanding of some of the basic problems involved in vascular penile circulation.

LDF is particularly useful for assessing the microcirculation of patients with diabetic microangiopathy, for detecting vasospasm caused by smoking or other vasospastic agents, and for studying the effects of various drugs in physiological and pathological conditions. There is convincing evidence that smoking is a major risk factor in the pathogenesis of both erectile dysfunction and vascular disease (Mikhailidis and Jeremy 1993). It is also known that there is a functional impairment of penile smooth muscle contractility and neurogenic relaxation in the corpus cavernosum of impotent men with abnormal penile hemodynamics. The so-called vasospasm or altered smooth muscle relaxation and responsiveness is likely to be a very important, but often temporary, factor in the etiology of erectile dysfunction. In fact penile microvascular disease is thought to be an important cause of erectile dysfunction and its presence is always suggested by a poor erectile response to cavernosal relaxant drugs such as papaverine (Virag et al. 1984). This situation is often present in patients suspected for a penile veno-occlusive dysfunction.

Whereas vasospasm is a temporary disorder that affects smooth muscle relaxation, penile diabetic microangiopathy is a chronic disease of patients with long-lasting diabetes and associated microvascular damage. In diabetic patients structural microvascular abnormalities are related to an increased blood flow which leads to capillary damage via increased capillary pressure (Parving et al. 1983). Abnormalities of capillary pressure regulation have been demonstrated in the nail fold of diabetic subjects during periods of poor glycemic control (Tooke 1983). Recent evidence suggests that capillary hypertension may be present in patients with diabetic nephropathy even when the hand is at heart level. According to hemodynamic hypothesis, raised capillary pressure stimulates the production of a thickened basement membrane and arteriolar sclerosis – ultrastructural hallmarks of diabetic microangiopathy. Early in the diabetic's life there is increased basal blood flow in kidney, retina, muscles, and skin; an impaired autoregulation is also apparent at this stage. As the diabetes progresses, blood flow decreases, resulting in underperfusion of retina, skin, renal, and other peripheral microvascular beds. When diabetic microangiopathy affects penile microcirculation, one also finds accelerated atherosclerosis of penile tissue and the increased presence of fibrotic lesions.

The development of LDF provides a noninvasive technique with which to examine blood flux (flow) in a superficial microvascular bed. Carefully applied LDF can provide a valuable, noninvasive assessment of the skin microcirculation and its control in diabetic subjects, heavy smokers, vascular patients, and patients undergoing pharmacological vasoactive therapy.

The aim of this chapter is to provide some basic information about the possible uses of LDF in the evaluation of normals, diabetics, heavy smokers, and vascular patients and in assessing therapies for erectile dysfunction. All the evaluations of penile microcirculation were performed using the LDF devices Periflux (Perimed, Sweden) and Laserflo (T.S.I., U.S.A.) with a laser light of 0.75 mm. Both of these LDFs permit the quantitative and qualitative evaluation of penile microcirculation. Microcirculatory flow values are expressed as milliliters per second per cubic centimeter of tissue. All flux values were obtained in a room at constant temperature ($22° \pm 1°C$).

Penile Microcirculation in Impotent Smokers

Penile blood flow and penile microcirculation were evaluated in 26 impotent heavy smokers (more than 15 cigarettes daily; Ledda et al. 1991). Their mean age was 46.6 years (range 28–66), and penile brachial index (PBI) was 0.79 (range 0.72–0.87) while smoking. Microcirculatory flow values were measured after 1 day and after 4 weeks without smoking cigarettes and again 10 min after smoking one cigarette (Table 1). The mean flow after 4 weeks without smoking was significantly greater (0.54 ml/min $\times$ 100 cm^3) than after 1 day without smoking. The mean microcirculatory flow 10 min after smoking one cigarette was significantly lower (0.32 ml/min $\times$ 100 cm^3). At the same time, flow pressure values obtained by color Doppler and plethysmography were remarkably better after 4 weeks without smoking, achieving PBI values from 0.75 to 0.92 (mean 0.83).

Table 1. Relationship between penile brachial index (PBI) and microcirculatory flow and smoking

	While smoking	After 1 day without smoking	After 4 weeks without smoking	10 Min after smoking 1 cigarette
PBI	0.72 – 0.87 (mean 0.79)	–	0.75 – 0.92 (mean 0.83)	–
Micro-circulatory flow[a]	0.30	0.42	0.54	0.32

PBI, Penile Brachial Index

[a] Microcirculatory flow is evaluated in ml/min $\times$ 100 cm^3 of tissue

Penile Skin Flux in Normals, Diabetics, and Vascular Patients

Fifty normal subjects, 50 diabetics, and 50 vascular patients (with intermittent claudication and a walking distance of 800–1500 m) were evaluated with the probe of LDF (Laserflo) placed on the distal dorsal third of the penis (A. Ledda, unpublished data). Twenty-five diabetic patients and 20 vascular patients had been referred for erectile dysfunction of varying degree. All subjects were injected with intracavernosal papaverine (8 mg, minitest) with a fine needle (0.30 mm). Microcirculatory measurements were obtained at 35 °C skin temperature (using a thermostat) and repeated at 45 °C (after 10 min heating). The skin flow increase upon thermic stimulation was also recorded. To compare skin flow variations with the cavernosal flow variation after papaverine and after thermal stimulation, the cavernosal flow was assessed with an intracavernosal needle probe in two normal subjects, three diabetics, and three vascular patients. (All statistical differences were assessed by the Mann-Whitney U test and by ANOVA). The three groups were similar in age distribution. The penile index (penile to arm pressure ratio) did not differ significantly between the two groups of patients (Table 2). There were also no differences in either age or penile index between those with and without impotence.

Table 2. Clinical data of normal subjects and patients. Mean values

		Normal subjects	Diabetics patients A	B	Vascular A	B
No.		50	25	25	30	20
Age	mean	51	52	51.1	52	52.2
	sd	9	8	7	8	8
Penile index		>1	0.8	0.72	0.7	0.72
SD			0.01	0.03	0.02	0.02

A, Not impotent
B, Impotent

Table 3. Penile skin flow (mean SD) in normal subjects, diabetics, and vascular patients

	Time (min)	Normal subjects	Diabetics patients	Vascular
Injection	0	0.53 (0.1)	0.76 (0.1)*	0.48 (0.08)
	5	2.88 (0.8)	1.06 (0.1)*	0.98 (0.1)*
	10	2.58 (0.7)	1.1 (0.3)*	1.68 (0.1)*
	15	2.33 (0.8)	0.93 (0.1)*	1.12 (0.2)*

* $p < 0.05$: difference from normal subjects

As presented in Table 3, there was a significant increase in skin flux among diabetics compared with normals in the resting state. There was also a significantly lower increase in flux in both groups of patients after 5, 10, and 15 min. However, the test was not able to differentiate between those with and those without impotence. The differences in measurements induced by local warming are shown in Table 4. Skin flux at 35 ° and 45 °C in both groups of patients was significantly lower than in normals. However, there were no significant differences between those with and those without impotence. In both the diabetic and the vascular group the flux increase after thermal stimulation was significantly lower than in normals, and it was lower in patients with impotence than in those without impotence (Fig. 1). Finally, Fig. 2 shows the variation in cavernosal flux after papaverine. The same differences were observed

Table 4. Penile skin flow at 35 ° and 40 °C in normal subjects and patients who are (B)/are not impotent (A)

	Normal subjects	Diabetics patients		Vascular	
		A	B	A	B
Flow at 35°	0.54 (0.1)	0.78 (0.1)	0.79 (0.1)	0.48 (0.07)	0.3 (0.05)
Flow at 45°	2.38 (0.7)	1.22 (0.3)	1.14 (0.1)	1.24 (0.33)	1.01 (0.1)
Difference	1.84 (0.9)	0.44 (0.1)	0.35* (0.08)	0.76 (0.1)	0.46* (0.1)

* $p < 0.05$: difference within the group (between patients with and without impotence)

Fig. 1. Skin flow difference before and after thermal stimulation

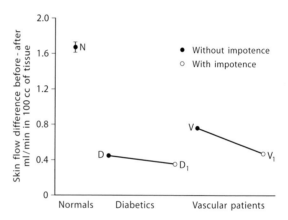

Fig. 2. Cavernosal flow (*cav*) evaluated by laser Doppler flowmetry after papaverine injection. *Nor*, normal; *Dia*, diabetic; *Vasc*, vascular patients

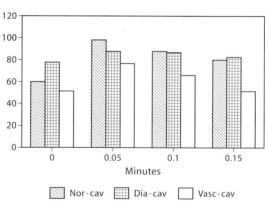

among the three groups as at baseline. However, cavernosal flux was at its peak in all three groups after 5 min while peak flux values after papaverine were observed in the skin after 10 min.

Conclusion

LDF proved very useful in assessing acute effects of smoking (studied 10 min after smoking one cigarette) and of the improvement of penile microcirculatory parameters after 4 weeks without smoking. The acute and chronic effects on penile microcirculation due to smoking are the result of a significant persistent vasospasm which can be completely reversed after 4 weeks without smoking. The results of a drug-induced erection test (cavernous pharmacological injection) may therefore be misleading. According to Glina et al. (1988), we can say that cigarette smoking can interfere, in fact, with any pharmacological diagnostic or therapeutic approach to erectile dysfunction. Furthermore, LDF showed interesting flux differences among normals, diabetics, and vascular patients. The differences were more significant after papaverine injection, which discriminated between patients and normals but not between those with and without erectile dysfunction.

It was also very important to observe that differences between patients with and those without erectile dysfunction were revealed by the thermal stimulation test even better than those obtained after intracavernous papaverine injection. The differences in skin flux were also observed and compared with intracavernosal measurement, as obtained by the laser-light-needle. Intracavernosal flux after papaverine showed an earlier peak (after 5 min) than peak skin flux (after 10 min). This suggests that studying penile skin flux we observed a proportionally reduced flux in comparison with cavernosal flux, but that the differences between normals and patients were comparable.

In conclusion, we can observe that LDF is useful in evaluating patients with suspected vasculogenic erectile dysfunction to monitor the effects of treatments (or of vasospastic agents) and to quantify skin (or cavernosal) flux changes following them. It can also be used to follow up the long-term course of diabetic microangiopathy and vascular disease.

References

Borgos (1994) Principles of instrumentation: calibration and technical issues. In: Laser Doppler. Med-Orion, London

Fagrell (1994) Problems using Laser Doppler on skin in clinical practice. In: Laser Doppler. Med-Orion, London

Glina S, Reichelt AC, Leao PP, Sos Reins JMSM (1988) Impact of cigarette smoking on papaverine-induced erection. J Urol 140:523-524

Ledda A, Tenaglia R, Belcaro C (1991) Laser Doppler flowmetry in impotent smokers. Arteres Veines 10:179-180

Mikhailidis DP, Jeremy JY (1993) Il ruolo delle prostaglandine nell'erezione e nell'impotenza. In: Andrologia vascolare. Minerva Medica, Turin

Parving HH, Viberti GC, Keen H, Christiansen JS, Lassen NA (1983) Haemodynamic factors in the genesis of diabetic microangiopathy. Metabolism 32:943

Tooke JE (1983) Capillary pressure in non-insulin-dependent diabetics. Int Ang 2(4):167

Virag R, Frydman D, Legman M, Virag H (1984) Intracavernous injection of papaverine as a diagnostic and therapeutic method in erectile failures. Angiology 35:79

Venous Leakage as a Cause of Erectile Failure: Myth or Reality?

J. A. VALE

Introduction

Although the concept that impotence might result from a failure of occlusion of venous channels from the penis was suggested as early as the turn of this century [1–3], venous leak surgery remains a highly controversial subject. The reasons for this are the varying success rate of venous leak surgery and the fact that pathological studies of "leaky veins" frequently show no discernible changes. Before considering the evidence for and against the concept of venous leakage, it is important to review the basic anatomy and physiology of venous mechanisms in the development of an erection.

Penile Venous Anatomy

Venous return from the erectile tissue of the pendulous portion of the penis occurs mainly through the deep dorsal vein of the penis. The blood from the endothelial-lined lacunar spaces of the corpora cavernosa reaches the deep dorsal vein by small venules that form the subtunical plexus, and they coalesce to form the emissary veins that penetrate the tunica albuginea. The deep dorsal vein is usually single, and has valves which prevent retrograde flow. It drains into Santorini's vesico-prostatic plexus and thus into the internal pudendal veins. There is also a superficial venous system of the penis, which drains mainly the skin and subcutaneous tissues and is highly variable in its termination. The proximal crura of the penis drain through the cavernous and crural veins, which also terminate in the internal pudendal veins.

Physiology of the Penile Venous System

In the flaccid penis the trabecular smooth muscle of the copora cavernosa is contracted, and venous drainage occurs relatively freely in a situation of low outflow resistance. During tumescence the cavernosal smooth muscle relaxes, permitting filling of the lacunar spaces with blood. The resulting rise in intracavernous pressure causes compression of the subtunical venous plexus against the tunica albuginea, increasing outflow resistance. As the intrapenile blood pressure increases towards systolic blood pressure, the penis becomes rigid, and this passive venous compression is maximal. At full erection the emissary veins are probably also occluded by stretching of the tunica albuginea. Obviously there must be some venous drainage during erection; otherwise there would be stasis, with ischaemia and ultimately priapism. Although compression of the subtunical and emissary veins is a passive phenomenon, the primary process leading to venous occlusion is relaxation of the trabecular smooth muscle of the corpora cavernosa. This smooth muscle relaxation is under the control of the cholinergic autonomic nerves derived from the pelvic neural plexus. Penile erection therefore represents an equilibrium between arterial inflow and venous outflow. Detumescence occurs when vasoconstrictive (probably adrenergic) impulses cause contraction of the arterial smooth muscle and the trabecular smooth muscle. This leads to a reduction in intracavernous pressure, and permits the subtunical and emissary veins to open.

Venous Leakage and Impotence

There can be no doubt that erectile failure can result from a failure of venous closure mechanisms. The evidence for this comes from physiological studies, in particular pharmacocavernosometry which demonstrates that in some patients a high infusion rate is required to produce and sustain an erection. This demonstrates a situation of low outflow resistance, which is clearly indicative of a failure of veno-occlusive mechanisms.

However, the suggestion that this is a primary venous problem is facile. Pathological studies of the veins of patients with venous leakage often show no discernible change, and if any change is noted it is usually one of fibrosis which may develop secondary to increased flow and pressure resulting from a failure of veno-occlusion [4]. The physiological features of venous incompetence could be produced if the trabecular smooth muscle did not relax normally, thus causing a failure of passive venous occlusion. Smooth muscle cell changes have been noted in the corpora cavernosa of some impotent patients, with fragmentation and loss of the basal lamina, nuclear changes and a reduction in contractile elements within the cytoplasm [5, 6], and a reduction in smooth muscle content has been measured objectively using computerised image analysis in patients with venous leakage [7]. Organ bath studies of cavernosal smooth muscle from patients with venous impotence have demonstrated a marked impairment of the normal relaxation response to electrical field stimulation [8]. Interestingly the relaxant response to papaverine was not significantly different from that of cavernosal muscle from control patients, suggesting that this may be a neurogenic/neurotransmitter failure.

Of course, it is possible that the aetiology of venogenic impotence may be multifactorial, with some patients having a primary trabecular smooth muscle problem and others having a true venous problem. For example, quite a high proportion of patients with impotence and Peyronie's disease appear to have a venous problem which may be related to the plaque rigidity, preventing normal venous closure mechanisms from operating. One very interesting study has shown that patients who have a normal single potential analysis of cavernous electrical activity (SPACE) and proven venous leakage have a good post-operative outcome from venous leak surgery, whilst patients with an abnormal single potential analysis of cavernous electrical activity do poorly [9]. Although SPACE and its significance remain highly controversial, SPACE abnormalities are believed to relate to pathology of the cavernosal smooth muscle or its neural supply. This suggests that patients with normal smooth muscle activity and venous leakage may represent a good prognostic group for venous leak surgery; their pathology may be one of primary venous disease. Further studies are necessary to elucidate this.

The Assessment of Venous Leakage

Radiological assessment of venous leakage really attempts to measure outflow resistance during an erection. Two techniques are commonly used: pharmacocavernosometry and colour Doppler imaging (CDI). As an initial step, both investigations require relaxation of the trabecular smooth muscle and arterial smooth muscle to mimic the conditions at the start of an erection. This is produced pharmacologically using papaverine or prostaglandin E_1. Pharmacocavernosometry then requires the infusion of normal saline using a carefully calibrated pump, in order that the infusion rate to generate and maintain an erection can be determined [10]. In a situation of low resistance and venous leakage the infusion rate to induce and maintain an erection is clearly higher than in a normal high-resistance situation. With CDI the maximal systolic flow velocity is determined to assess arterial function, and the minimum diastolic velocity is used to assess outflow resistance [11]. A relatively high minimum diastolic velocity suggests low resistance and venous leakage, and a resistance index can be determined (Fig. 1).

Although there are proponents of both methods of evaluation of venous leakage, the use of CDI is fundamentally flawed in my opinion. Patients with significant venous leakage do not achieve erection with papaverine or prostaglandin E_1, and if there is no full erection, one cannot possibly comment on a passive veno-occlusive mechanism which requires full rigidity for its operation. The most information that CDI can yield is the suspicion of a venous leak if the maximum systolic velocities are normal in the absence of an erection. The patient still requires

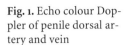

Fig. 1. Echo colour Doppler of penile dorsal artery and vein

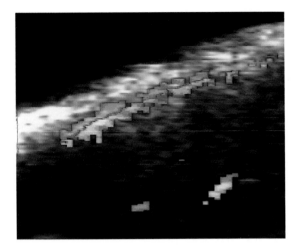

pharmacocavernosometry to confirm the diagnosis, and pharmacocavernosometry also has the advantage that contrast medium can be infused via the cannula, thus permitting localisation of the incompetent veins.

In my opinion the only role for CDI in the assessment of venous leak patients is to establish that there is no evidence of an arteriogenic problem. This is clearly mandatory if venous leak surgery is contemplated, and some of the disappointing results of venous leak surgery in early series may have been due to the inclusion of patients with primary arteriogenic or mixed vascular pathology.

Should We Perform Venous Leak Surgery?

There are really two arguments against venous leak surgery. The first is that venous leakage does not exist as a primary condition and is a consequence of a change in trabecular smooth muscle function, as discussed above. The idea, therefore, that tying off some of the veins from the penis would make any difference is simplistic and flawed. However, in my opinion, this argument is overstated. Firstly, the work of Stief et al. [9] with SPACE suggests that there may be some patients in whom the primary problem is a defect in subtunical or intratunical venous compression. These patients may reasonably be expected to benefit from venous leak surgery. Secondly, although venous leak surgery may not address the primary pathology in those patients who have an abnormality of the trabecular smooth muscle function, the aim of surgery is to increase venous resistance. Although this does not address the primary pathology, it may nonetheless achieve the desired physiological effect. There are many other examples in surgical practice of such a principle, including all types of bypass surgery.

With regard to the argument that the long-term results of venous leak surgery are poor, I have recently examined the results of venous leak surgery in a carefully selected group of patients with normal arterial function proven on CDI [12]. All patients underwent venous leak surgery using a standardised approach in which the deep dorsal vein of the penis was excised and ligated, and any large accessory veins were also removed. One year after surgery 64% of patients were able to have sexual intercourse, although one-third of these required papaverine or prostaglandin self-injection. None of these patients had been able to have intercourse with or without papaverine prior to surgery, and when asked whether they would undergo the procedure again, 65% responded positively. Interestingly, patients responding positively were not necessarily those who had a favourable outcome from surgery, illustrating the point that these patients are frequently desperate and are willing to try any measure that may restore potency. Given an operating time of only 30–60 min, a very low complication rate, and the opportunity to perform venous leak surgery as a day case, I believe that venous leak surgery is worthwhile in properly selected patients who are fully informed prior to surgery. After all, the only other options open to these patients are the use of a vacuum device or insertion of a penile prosthesis.

References

1. Duncan JA (1895) Old age – a myth. Toledo Med Surg Reporter 3:163–164
2. Wotton JA (1902) Ligation of the dorsal vein of the penis as a cure for atonic impotence. Texas Med J 18:325–328
3. Lydstone GF (1908) The surgical treatment of impotency. Am J Clin Med 15:1571–1573

4. Hirsch M, Lubestsky R, Goldman H, Agarwal V, Melman A (1993) Dorsal vein sclerosis as a predictor of outcome in penile venous ligation surgery. J Urol 150:1810–1813

5. Persson C, Diederisch W, Lue TF, Benedict Yen TS, Fishman IJ, McLin PH, Tanagho EA (1989) Correlation of altered penile ultrastructure with clinical arterial evaluation. J Urol 142:1462–1468

6. Jevitch MJ, Khawand NY, Vidic B (1990) Clinical significance of ultrastructural findings in the corpora cavernosa of normal and impotent men. J Urol 143:289–293

7. Wespes E, Goes PM, Shiffmann S, Depierreux M, Vanderhaeghen JJ, Schulman CC (1991) Computerized analysis of smooth muscle fibers in potent and impotent patients. J Urol 146:1015–1017

8. Pickard RS, King P, Zar MA, Powell PH (1994) Corpus cavernosal relaxation in impotent men. Br J Urol 74:485–491

9. Stief CG, Djamiliaan M, Truss MC, Tan H, Thon WF, Jonas U (1984) Prognostic factors for the postoperative outcome of penile venous surgery for venogenic erectile dysfunction. J Urol 151:880–883

10. Eardley I, Vale JA, Holmes S, Patel A, Kirby RS, Lumley JSP (1990) Pharmacocavernometry in the assessment of erectile impotence. J Roy Soc Med 83:22–25

11. Patel U, Amin Z, Friedman E, Vale J, Kirby RS, Lees WR (1993) Colour flow and spectral Doppler imaging after papaverine-induced penile erection in 220 impotent men: study of temporal patterns and the importance of repeated sampling, velocity asymmetry and vascular anomalies. Clin Radiol 48:18–24

12. Vale JA, Feneley MR, Lees WR, Kirby RS (1995) Venous leak surgery: long term follow up of patients undergoing excision/ligation of the deep dorsal vein of the penis. Br J Urol 76:192–195

Medical Treatment of Erectile Dysfunction

G.F. Menchini Fabris, P. Cilurzo, P.M. Giorgi, and P. Turchi

Introduction

Since the beginning of civilization man has always tried to improve his sexual potency. Each culture has had its own beliefs about the aphrodisiac properties, real or imaginary, attributed to certain plants, mushrooms, animal extracts, cocktails of spices, and exotic foods. Folklore and religions have attributed medicinal properties to some of these substances, occasionally with some biological basis. These substances can still easily be found today and are sometimes used, for example, ginseng (*Panax* genus). The coca leaves that are chewed by the Incas to increase their physical strength and endurance while working in the mines have been shown to be a sexual stimulant. The effects of cocaine are among the strongest regarding ability and intensity during sexual relations.

The most widely used sexual stimulants in Africa, the Orient, and central South America are marihuana and hashish while those in Europe are spices, for example, ginger, pepper, parsley, cucumber, squash seeds, cantharis, celery, and asparagus, which produce irritation or a burning sensation in the urogenital tract. On the basis of their effects aphrodisiacs can be subdivided into three groups: (a) those with a general invigorating effect (alkaloids including strychnine, yohimbine, etc.), (b) those with a central disinhibiting effect (e.g., amphetamines, alcohol), and (c) those with a stimulating effect on the urogenital zone (e.g., cantharidin in powder form obtained by dehydrating the *Lytta vesicatoria* coleopter).

Aside from these historic and anecdotal aspects, there is also a well-defined scientific study regarding the use and efficiency of certain recognized drugs in the medicinal therapy of male sexual erectile dysfunction. However, it is often the case that the concept of the patient's sexual health at the basis of the medical treatment for male sexual erectile dysfunction becomes reduced to giving him a "better erection" (the final mechanical stage of male excitement) rather than correcting the cause of the problem.

Medical Therapy for Male Sexual Erectile Dysfunction

In 1849 Berthold [1] first observed that the testicles produce a substance that is responsible for sexual behavior in the rooster. These first observations are considered the beginning of experimental endocrinology. Since then numerous scientific studies have confirmed that the male sexual drive, in all known existing mammalian species, is androgen dependent. The role of testosterone begins during the intrauterine stage; it regulates sexual differentiation by means of the action that it exerts at the diencephalic level (hypothalamic impregnation) and at the peripheral level (the external genitalia). In the adult testosterone continues to play an essential role in the reproductive cycle. It controls sexual behavior (desire); it influences the erectile mechanism, the development of the genitalia; and it plays an essential role in spermatogenesis. Hypogonadism is closely related to the plasma testosterone level and spontaneous (nocturnal erections) or provoked sexual activity. In subjects who have experienced a normal development and sex life, the cortical component becomes dominant over the hormonal tone. For example, in the case of a marked reduction in testosterone levels, such as after chemical or surgical castration [2], there is no sudden reduction in sexual potency. On the basis of these observations, therapy with testosterone or its derivatives has been widely used, with very satisfying results, in cases of male sexual erectile dysfunction resulting from a primary testicular hypofunctioning or due to an insufficient hypothalamic-hypophysis stimulation (real hypogonadism with reduced levels of testosterone). The treatment of male sexual erectile dysfunction with androgens, in the presence of normal endogenous circulating levels of testosterone, is not usually effective, other than causing an increased libido.

The "depot" forms of testosterone (cypionate, propionate, enanthate, etc.) are administered by intramuscular injections every 2–4 weeks.

Generally these are well tolerated; however, the patient must be closely monitored for adverse side effects, such as impaired hepatic function and/or marked prostatic hypertrophy or metaplasia. Testosterone or its derivatives may be administered during puberty only when there exists a true condition of hypogonadism, and then only for short periods and under strict supervision. Testosterone is administered orally, which has the advantage of being less toxic due to its reduced hepatic metabolism; however, this has less therapeutic effect than the deposit forms. Mesterolone, with an action similar to that of dihydrotestosterone, can also be administered orally; but at the dosage normally used this drug has very little effect on libido and sexual potency.

When hormonal deficiency is responsible for reduced gonadotropic stimulation on the Leydig's cells or reduced receptor response even in the presence of normal levels of luteinizing hormone (LH), the patient can be started on human chorionic gonadotropin (hCG), which acts on LH. Normal plasma levels of LH may even obscure quantitative and/or qualitative alterations in pituitary secretions. In the former case there is an immunologically apparently normal level of LH molecules, but in reality it has a limited biological activity; in the latter case there may be an altered timing of the release of GnRH, thereby inappropriately producing plasma peaks of LH. In all of these cases the treatment of choice is hCG. This is because it maintains a normal gonadal tropism, in contrast to treatment with testosterone or its derivatives, which are partially reduced by a negative feedback at the central level. In addition, the androgenic secretory response is self-limiting due to the phenomena of down-regulation. The plasma levels of testosterone are more physiological than those obtained by the direct administration of androgens [3].

A particular use for hCG is in the treatment of male sexual impotency due to chronic renal insufficiency. In these cases the hypothesis is that there is a reduced biological activity of endogenous LH, with an analogous reduction in the levels of testosterone and dihydrotestosterone. The administration of hCG has been shown to reestablish plasma testosterone levels to a point allowing a return to normal sexual function [4].

Dopaminergic deficiency in the male can manifest itself by hyperprolactinemia and erectile dysfunction, which are related to a functional alteration in the hypothalmic-pituitary-gonadal axis. In these cases the recovery of normal sexual function is secondary to restorating control of prolactin secretion by dopaminergic drugs such as bromocryptine. Finally, when the sexual disorder is part of an endocrine syndrome (hypothyroidism, cortisol deficiency, etc.) or of metabolic diseases such as diabetes, the physician must first treat these underlying problems.

Transdermal Treatment

A recent addition to the possible therapeutic modalities for treating male sexual erectile dysfunction has been the transdermal administration of medication. This method is one of the oldest means of administering drugs in the history of medicine. One need only think of how long cataplasms, compresses, etc. have been used. In modern medicine this method was initially used exclusively in the field of dermatology, but today it is slowly being introduced and accepted in various other fields. Today, for example, the use of nitroglycerin patches to treat ischemic heart disease or patches with estrogen to treat postmenopausal syndromes represent therapeutic reality. In recent years transdermal therapy has also been evaluated in the area of andrology. For example, it has been proposed to use patches containing testosterone for the therapy of primary hypogonadism [5], and dihydrotestosterone in the form of an alcoholic gel for that of prepubertal gynecomastia in males [6, 7]. In recent years the medical treatment of male sexual erectile dysfunction has undergone a virtual cultural revolution, with the advent of intracavernosal administration of vasoactive drugs (papaverine, phentolamine, prostaglandin, etc.) for penile erectile dysfunction. This technique has enabled the physician to make great strides in understanding the pathophysiology of an erection and the treatment of male sexual potency problems [8].

We have witnessed such dramatic changes in the treatment of sexual problems that there now exists the possibility of local or topical treatment along with other types of therapy, for example, the hormonal. However, there are a number of undesirable side effects and complications (e.g., painful injections, priapism, cavernitis, fibrosis, ecchymosis) that may result from intracavernosal therapy, and these are often associated with decreased cooperation on the part of the patient with this treatment, which involves repeated injections. Transdermal treatments may therefore assume a more important role in the administration of vasoactive medication, as well as other compounds that have a specific action on the penile corpus cavernosum.

From a strictly pharmacokinetic standpoint two pathways can be distinguished in the absorption of transdermal medication: passive and active. Passive absorption occurs exclusively on the basis of the physicochemical properties of the molecular structure of the drug, in particular the degree of liposolubility and the concentration gradient between cutaneous and the subcutaneous surfaces. Active absorption takes place through the use of applied energy, specifically that produced by an electrical field, capable of inducing an accelerated active transport [9, 10]. This method is known as iontophoresis, or the controlled transdermal drugs administration system. We have tried both passive and active transdermal administration of two substances that have an effect on erectile dynamics: yohimbine and papaverine hydrochloride. Yohimbine, an indole alkaloid with α_2-blocking action, has been used in the past as an aphrodisiac. Even today its actual pharmacological action on adrenergic receptors is not well characterized. It has an activating effect on the central mechanisms or a localized action at the level of the penile cavernosum [11, 12]. Papaverine has a muscle-relaxing effect on the pariarteriolar smooth muscle fibrils, which causes a filling of the vascular lacunae in the cavernosal tissue initially by means of an active mechanism and subsequently by a passive reduction in the venous return in the penile venous system, given its particular anatomic position under the tunica albuginea.

To allow its administration by the passive intradermal method yohimbine was prepared in ointment form at a concentration of 5%, in an oil/water type of emulsion using isopropyl lanolin as the excipient. This study was conducted in a group of 62 patients at various degrees of sexual erectile dysfunction, as determined from patient history, objective examination, measurement of hormonal levels, dynamic flow measurements, and nocturnal penile tumescence test. These patients were given alternate doses of medication and a comparable placebo (cross-over trial) design. During this trial blood samples were taken from the cavernosal tissue to establish a pharmacokinetic drug absorption curve. The results show an effective passage of the medication to the inside of the corpus cavernosum. Maximum absorption values were obtained about 25 min after the medication was applied, with an average concentration level of about 58 ng/ml.

Clinically there was both qualitative and quantitative improvement in the dynamics of penile erection among those with an average degree of erectile deficiency that was of recent onset. This clinical impression was confirmed by statistical comparison using the information obtained from diaries that the patients themselves kept during the entire period of treatment. They recorded the frequency and quality of their sexual en-coun-ters, with the data obtained while they were taking the placebo.

Our experience in the active transdermic administration of papaverine hydrocloride derives from iontophoresis (controlled transdermal drugs administration system). This technique is not new and it has been pre-viously used for the treatment of many pathological conditions in other fields of medicine. Although it was known as early as 1747 by Veratti, it was only at the beginning of the twentieth century that Leduc showed, in a clear and precise manner, the possibility of using iontophoresis as a means of transporting polarized medications by means of an electric current across a cutaneous barrier [10]. This became the method of choice for the administration of pilocarpine for the laboratory diagnosis of cystic fibrosis, and it was also used in the treatment of cutaneous hyperhydrosis, the symptomatic therapy of trigeminal neuralgia, and cu-taneous anesthesia with lidocaine.

In practice, a small electric generator produces a continuous electric current, fed by a nickel-cadmium battery, which provides the energy for the creation of an electric field capable of inducing the migration of polarized medication through the skin when the electric circuit is closed. In our case we used papaverine hydrochloride (PaCL) because this salt is extremely water soluble, and under the effect of a continuous current it easily undergoes dielectrolysis, disassociating into papaverine and Cl^{2-} ions. Once the iontophoretic circuit is closed, a saturated force field is created that induces the migration of positively charged ions to penetrate the epidermis migrating towards the anode, while the negatively charged ions move toward the cathode. This creates an active transdermal accel-erated transport system. In practice, this system can be influenced by numerous other factors due to the interaction of the electric current with the tissues and other biological structures.

PaCL, diluted in double-distilled H_2O at a concentration of 20 mg/ml was placed into a cylindrical electrode of a size large enough to accom-modate the penis. The electrode especially prepared for this purpose was constructed from a conducting plastic resin and designed so as to permit the greatest possible contact between the cutaneous surface of the penis and the solution containing papaverine. Included in these therapeutic trials were 26 patients who had undergone a cycle of iontophoretic treatments [6], one treatment per week. Each treatment consisted of the following; an electric current of 6.0–8.0 mA, lasting 20 min, with a volume of 140 ml PaCL at a concentration of 20 mg/ml. A series of samples of papaverine hydrochloride were taken before and after each treatment, and these were tested by chromatography using thin sheets of silica gel.

The laboratory results showed a reduction in the concentration of the medication during each treatment equal to 10.3% ± 2.7%. Eleven patients (42.3%) showed a clinical improvement in sexual activity, with a marked improvement in the quality of erection, an increase in the time that it was maintained, and an increase in the frequency of sexual encounters. Obviously, during the treatments the patients never had an erection however, tumescence and a slight transitory hyperemia of the skin and mucous membrane were noted. These symptoms were not accompanied by any painful sensation on the skin or the external urethral orifice of the penis. In terms of clinical evaluation we conclude that there was a net improvement in the condition of these patients with a mild grade of vascular deficiency, including diabetics and subjects who smoked.

Effects of Systemic Treatment

Hypotensive Drugs

Numerous drugs commonly used to treat arterial hypertension can produce erectile dysfunction (Table 1). Clonidine, an active drug (excitatory) that affects the α-adrenergic centers of the CNS (diencephalon) depresses arterial pressure by the interaction on the vascular receptors. In the genitals, this can be the cause of an erectile deficiency. α-Methyldopa, an adrenergic mediator, can also reduce sexual potency. The β-blocking drugs used especially for adolescent hypertension and for hyperthyroidism and tachyarrhythmias can also cause erectile dysfunction depending on the dosage and the duration of the treatment. Reserpine, used much less frequently today, is often prescribed in conjunction with diuretics

Table 1. Categories of drugs and specific agents causing erectile dysfunction

Antihypertensive drugs	Clonidine
	α-Methyldopa
	β-Blockers
	Reserpine
Gastrointestinal drugs	Cimetidine
	Ranitidine
	Metoclopramide
	Domperidone
Dermatological drugs	Ketaconazole
Anti-inflammatory drugs	Steroids
Anabolic drugs	Androgenic drugs
Antineoplastic drugs	All
Psychotherapeutic drugs	Sulpiride
	Amitiptyline
	Fluoxetine
	Alprazolam
	Maprolidine

and/or vasodilators and can cause hyperprolactinemia, with a reduction of the libido and sexual potency.

Antiulcer and Gastrokinetic Drugs

The compounds used in gastroenterology to treat gastroduodenitis and peptic ulcers are antagonists of the H_2 histamine receptors (cimetidine, ranitidine, nizaditine); in a small number of cases these cause sexual erectile dysfunction due to hyperprolactinemia (occasionally with gynecomastia) and a decrease in libido. Numerous gastrokinetic compounds that act on the filling function and gastric peristalsis, in particular metoclopramide, can also cause hyperprolactinemia. This side effect can be found even with the use of modest but prolonged doses of medication. Domperidone, despite the fact that it does not pass the blood-brain barrier as does metoclopramide, acts on the adenohypophysis stimulating the secretion of prolactin.

Psychotherapeutic Drugs

The sulpride is responsible for hyperprolactinemia even when used in small doses. A decrease in libido, erectile dysfunction, followed by gynecomasty and obesity are sometimes noted. Amitriptyline has an important effect of the endocrine system (even this drug produces hyperprolactinemia) as do other more recent compounds such as fluoxetine, maprotiline, and other benzodiazepines, which after long periods of treatment reduce the libido.

Dermatological Drugs

Ketoconazole, commonly used to treat cutaneous mycoses can, if used in topical form (cream, lotions, etc.) and especially if taken orally for a prolonged period, interfere with the production of steroids produced by the Leydig's cells, resulting in a decreased production rate of testosterone.

Anti-inflammatory Drugs

All steroid-based anti-inflammatory drugs exert a strong interference on the delicate sexual endocrine equilibrium of the diencephalon-pituitary-gonad system. In patients treated with cortisone-based medications for long periods an endocrine imbalance with hypogonadism and erectile dysfunction may arise. In addition, the corticosteroids have an important action on the prostate, favoring hypertrophy of the gland and prostatitis. These pathologies have a direct negative influence on sexual performance.

Anabolic Drugs

Anabolic drugs are commonly used without proper medical supervision, particularly in sports. The anabolic androgenic steroids are also used in the treatment of osteoporosis. The administration of these androgens initially creates a deregulating alteration in the pituitary-gonadal axis. In addition, the androgens, besides reducing the function of the gonadotrophins can produce prostatic alterations that have negative repercussions on sexual function.

Antineoplastic Drugs

Among the many side effects resulting from the use of antineoplastic medication is a reduction of the libido and erectile dysfunction. All the drugs used to combat neoplasms can be responsible for cytotoxic effects which can damage the gonads and reduce the production of testosterone, resulting in a decrease in libido and erectile dysfunction.

References

1. Berthold A (1849) Transplantation der Hoden. Arch Anat Physiol Wiss Med Berlin 42-46
2. Sachs BD, Meisel RL(1988) The physiology of male sexual behavior. In: Knobil E, Neill JD (eds) The physiology of reproduction. Raven, New York
3. Niesclagh E, Behere HM (eds) (1990) Testosterone: action, deficiency, substitution. Springer, Berlin Heidelberg New York
4. Menchini Fabris GF, Turchi P, Giorgio PM, Canale D(1990) Diagnosis and treatment of sexual dysfunction in patients affected by chronic renal failure on hemodialysis. In: D'Amico G, Colasanti G (eds) Contribution to nephrology. Karger, Basel, pp24-33
5. Bals-Prash M, Longer K, Place VA, Nieschlag (1988) Substitution therapy of hypogonadal men with transdermal testosterone over one year. Acta Endocrinol 118:7-11

6. Kuhn JM, Laudat MH, Roca R, Dugue MA, Luton JP, Bricarie H (1983) Gyneco-masties: effect du traitment prolongé par la dihydrotestosterone parvoie percuta-née. Press Med 12:21-27
7. Turchi P, Giorgi PM, Canale D, Menchini Fabris GF (1989) Attualità in andrologia e ginecologia. Adipoe ginecomastia. SES ediz., Naples, pp173-182
8. Brindley GS (1983) Cavernosal α blockade: a new technique for investigating and treating erectile impotence. Br J Psychiat 143:332
9. Banga AK, Chien YW (1988) Iontophoretic delivery of drugs: fundamentals, de-velopments and biomedical applications. J Controlled Release 7:1-24
10. Leduc S (1900) Introduction of medical substance into the depth of tissues by electric current. Ann d'electrobiol 3:545-560
11. Canale D, Cilurzo P, Turchi P, Bartelloni M, Giorgio PM, Menchini Fabris GF (1991) La terapia transdermica in andrologia. In: Pisani E, Austoni E (eds) Andro-logia '91. Monduzzi, Bologna, pp 401-407
12. Turchi P, Canale D, Ducci M, Nannipieri R, Serafini MF, Menchini Fabris GF (1992) The use of yohimbine in the transdermal treatment of male sexual im-potence. Int J Imp Res

Intracavernosal Drug Therapy

A. Ledda

Introduction

Intracavernosal pharmacotherapy became popular between 1982 and 1983 when Virag [14] and Brindley [3] demonstrated that injection of papaverine, phentolamine, and phenoxybenzamine into the cavernosal body induces a penile erection. One year later Virag [15] proposed a therapeutic protocol based on "self-injection". Patients suffering from penile erectile deficiency were examined, and those who showed a favorable response to intracavernous injections of papaverine were taught a technique that provides a "self-erection". Zorgniotti and Lefleur [17] in 1985 proposed a combination of papaverine and phentolamine, and immediately thereafter the use of prostaglandin E_1 (PGE_1) became a common practice. This drug was preferred over the others because of its lower rate of side effects, prolonged erections, and priapism than that with papaverine or papaverine + phentolamine. Today the use of these drugs has become routine, and constitutes either singularly or in combination the first step of every therapeutic protocol that deals with erectile dysfunction.

Intracavernous Injections: Materials and Methods

Any therapy must be preceded by a complete work-up of the patient. Erectile dysfunction can often be a warning sign for a more serious underlying pathological condition, and the physician confronting a patient with this problem must therefore conduct a general evaluation of the patient with particular attention to the vascular system. In 75% of cases the organic erectile dysfunction is secondary to some type of vasculopathy that can involve the arteries, veins, and microcirculation. These three vascular components are interrelated and cannot be separated; therefore the physician cannot diagnose an arteriogenic erectile deficiency or a veno-occlusive cavernosal pathology without knowing whether the microcirculation is intact, and whether it is affected by an acquired or congenital pathology.

Papaverine is used today in combination with phentolamine and/or PGE$_1$. Papaverine is metabolized in the liver and produces an elevated incidence of complications, specifically, prolonged erections, and priapism. Another complication derived from papaverine that must be considered is the extremely high incidence of fibrosis of the cavernosal bodies. Abozeid et al. [1] in 1987 found fibrosis in simian penile tissue submitted to chronic papaverine treatment. In 1984 Virag [15] proposed a "maxi-test" consisting of 80 mg papaverine.

Medication is not the only factor that can provide a certain level of intracavernosal pressure. Numerous other factors can distort the test results as well as the outcome of therapeutic self-injection. For example, the same dose of medication injected while the patient is under anesthesia induces a higher intracavernosal pressure; the reason for this is the lack of inhibiting factors that are usually present when the patient is in a conscious state, such as anxiety, which lead to the release of catecholamine and counteracts the action of the vasodilators.

Phentolamine is an α-blocker that is well tolerated by the cavernosal tissue and in combination with papaverine permits the use of smaller quantities of medication. This in turn reduces the incidence of prolonged erections and the risk of fibrosis in the corpus cavernosum. The pharmacological synergism is even more evident when PGE$_1$ is combined with papaverine and phentolamine. PGE$_1$ has the advantage over other compounds used in intracavernosal therapy of being almost completely metabolized in the corpus cavernosum and entailing a very low incidence of prolonged erections. A 5- to 6-year follow-up of 3200 patients showed no signs of fibrotic reactions caused by the PGE$_1$ [9]. The unfavorable aspects of PGE$_1$ are its high cost and postinjection pain (in 5%–10% of patients).

Other substances able to relax smooth muscle tissue have long been studied, and recently it was proposed to use a compound capable of producing nitric oxide (NO), the most well known among which is linsidomine chlorhydrate (SIN-1). However, since there is no clinical proof of the reliability of these substances, for the time being they cannot be used. On a practical level papaverine is no longer used alone due to its numerous undesirable side effects and particularly the risk of inducing fibrosis of the cavernosal tissue. Normally the therapy consists of: (a) 5–20 µg PGE_1, (b) 15 mg papaverine + 0.5 mg phentolamine, (c) 10 mg papaverine + 0.5 mg phentolamine + 10 µg PGE_1. Each patient has his own "personalized" medication or ideal combination of drugs. The initial injections, while containing the same dose of medication, can produce markedly different results regarding duration and quality of the erection. Eventually the self-injection therapy produces a more stable and uniform reaction to the drug.

Self-Injections and Intermittent Injections

Intracavernosal pharmacotherapy can be performed in two substantially different ways. Self-injection therapy offers the possibility, if the subject responds, of obtaining a pharmacological erection whenever he wishes to have sexual activity. It is therefore a real alternative therapy because it substitutes a chain of neurovascular reactions with a drug. The second possibility is that of using a pharmaceutical prosthesis in the form of intermittent injections or a closed therapeutic cycle that permits a functional recovery of the cavernosal body, which offers the patient the possibility of recovering a spontaneous erection without the use of self-injection therapy.

Our results in 2450 patients (average age, 48 years) over the past 8 years were evaluated after an initial cycle of 8 injections (performed by the patient himself) that covered a period of about 3 months. The first two injections were separated by 7 days, and the rest at intervals of about 15 days. The doses were individualized. At the conclusion of the cycle 65% of patients showed complete recovery of penile erection as early as the first injection; nevertheless the therapy was continued up to the last injection, if possible. Patients who abruptly interrupted the self-injection therapy protocol after the first 2–3 doses showed a high incidence of relapses; those who completed the entire cycle showed better recovery. Thirty percent of the patients continued the self-injection therapy despite the fact there was no sign of a spontaneous erection even after the second trimester of the protocol. Of the remaining 5% of patients ($n=120$) 60% ($n=72$) abandoned all types of therapy, and 40% ($n=48$) accepted the implantation of a penile prosthesis. It is important to point out that only patients who had a normal or dubious response to the diagnostic pharmacological erection tests were accepted for the pharmacological injection therapy, while patients who had either a serious case of fibrosis or a pathological response to the PGE_1 test, followed by and combined with a poor response of the penile echo color Doppler, were directed to a prosthesis implantation.

Conclusion

Eight years' experience with intracavernous injections has lead us to increasing belief in the potential of this therapy [5,9]. The first step before any therapy can be initiated is the elimination of any factors that can cause spasms of the smooth muscle and/or vasospasms in the penile microcirculation. This assumes that the patient has stopped smoking cigarettes, that anxiety has been attenuated by pharmacological and/or psychotherapeutic means, and that conditions such as diabetes, hypertension, and dislipidemia are kept under continuous control. The better the patient's general vascular condition, the greater is the potential of pharmacological therapy with intracavernosal injections [5-7, 9-13, 17].

The andrologist is first a physician, and therefore he cannot limit himself to providing the patient more rigidity to a flaccid penis but must identify all the factors contributing to the erectile dysfunction. In 1989 Conti and Virag [4] showed that the smooth musculature of the corpera cavernosa diminishes with age. While it is not yet possible to rejuvenate the patient, it is possible to slow down the process of vascular degeneration. The concept of ultrasonic arterial biopsy [2] or the vascular classification of the patient on the basis of an evaluation of the arterial walls should be remembered even when the physician treats a patient who will undoubtedly be proposed for penile prosthetic implant (Fig. 1, Table 1).

This is because, while it is correct to resolve the penile problem, it remains a professional obligation to attempt to prevent a heart attack and any other vascular pathology.

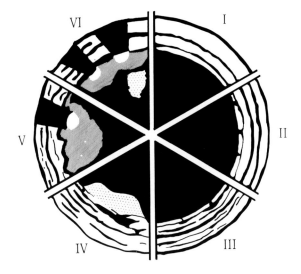

Fig. 1. Noninvasive ultrasonic biopsy

Table 1. Criteria for defining ultrasonic biopsy classes

	Description	Score[a]
I	Three layers, clearly separated (intima media and adventitia)	0
II	Initial intimal alterations, fatty streaks, intima media discontinuity and irregularity; unclear separation between walls (particularly intima media)	2
III	Microcalcifications, intima media granulation, early plaques (< 2mm)	4
IV	Plaques (> 2mm)	6
V	Plaques causing stenosis > 50%	8
VI	Plaques + stenosis associated with signs/symptoms (cardiac, peripheral and/or cerebral)	10

[a] Score relative to one artery. The ultrasonic biopsy score is the total score of two femoral + two carotids. The subjects' ultrasonic biopsy class is the class of the worst lesion among the four arterial sites evaluated.

References

1. Abozeid M, Juenemann KP, Luo J, et al (1987) Chronic papaverine treatment: the effect of repeated injections on the simian erectile response and penile tissue. J Urol 138:1263–1266
2. Belcaro G, Fisher C, Veller M et al (1993) Screening asymptomatic subjects with subclinical arteriosclerotic lesions with arterial ultrasonic biopsy. The PAP study. VASA 22/23:232–240
3. Brindley GS (1983) Cavernosal alpha-blockade: a new technique for investigating and treating erectile impotence. Br J Psychiatry 143:332
4. Conti G, Virag R (1989) Human penile erection and organic impotence. Normal hystology and hystopathology. In: Mayor G (ed) Urologia internationalis, vol 44. Karger, Basel, pp303–308
5. Ledda A, Seccia M, Martegiani C, Tenaglia R (1988) 18 mesi di esperienze con le farmacoprotesi peniene. Presented at the 61st Congress of the SIU, Cagliari, 20–23 September
6. Levine S, Althof SE, Turner LA, Risen CB et al (1989) Side effects of self-administration of intracavernous papaverine and phentolamine fore the treatment of impotence. J Urol 141:54
7. Lue TF, Tanagho EA (1987) Physiology of erection and pharmacological management of impotence. J Urol 137:829
8. Michal V, Kramar R, Pospichal J, Hejhol L (1977) Arterial epigastricocavernous anastomosis for the treatment of sexual impotence. World J Surg 1:515
9. Porst H (1994) Ten years of experience with various vasoactive drugs. Comparative studies in over 4000 patients. Int J Impotence Res 6 [Suppl 1]:D149
10. Saenz de Tejada I, Goldstein I, Azadzoi K, Krane RJ et al (1998) Impaired neurogenic and endothelium-mediated relaxation of arterial smooth muscle from diabetic men with impotence. N Engl J Med 320:1025
11. Sidi A, Cameron J, Duffy L, ND Lange P (1986) Intracavernous drug-induced erections in the management of male erectile dysfunction: experience with 100 patients. J Urol 135:704
12. Sidi A, Reddy P, Chen K (1988) Patient acceptance of and satisfaction with vasoactive intracavernous pharmacotherapy for impotence. J Urol 140:293
13. Stackl W, Hasun R, Merberger M (1988) Intracavernous injection of prostaglandin E_1 in impotent men. J Urol 140:66–68
14. Virag (1982) Intracavernous injection of papaverine for erectile failure. Letter to the Editor. Lancet 2:938
15. Virag (1984) Intracavernous injection of papaverine as a diagnostic and therapeutic method in erectile failure. Angiology 35:79/87
16. Virag R, Adaikan PG (1987) Effects of prostaglandin E_1 on penile erection and erectile failure. J Urol 139:1010
17. Zorgniotti AW, Lefleur RS (1988) Auto-injection of the corpus cavernosum with a vasoactive drug combination for vasculogenic impotence. J Urol 133:39–41

Surgical Treatment

G. Carmignani, S. De Stefani, and M. Capone

Surgical Treatment of Vasculogenic Erectile Dysfunction

The association between erectile dysfunction and decreased arterial flow deficiency to the corpus cavernosum was demonstrated for the first time by Leriche in 1923 [1]. He described a clinical syndrome characterized by claudication in the lower limbs, gluteal pain, and erectile dysfunction in a patient affected with an obstruction at the bifurcation of the iliac artery of an atherosclerotic nature. It was not until many years later that this association was correlated with an insufficient blood supply to the pelvic area and consequently to the corpus cavernosum. Since then much progress has been made in both the diagnostic and the therapeutic fields concerning erectile dysfunction, for example, with the discovery of vasoactive substances. When injected inside the corpus cavernosum of subjects without vascular alterations these provoke an erection similar to that occurring physiologically due to sexual excitement. These drugs, along with digital arteriographs, echo color Doppler, nocturnal penile tumescence test, and dynamic cavernosometry, have initiated a new era in the functional study of the vascularization of the penis and in the understanding of the pathophysiology of the erectile mechanism.

At the same rate, techniques have also been evolving for the reconstruction of adequate blood flow inside the corpus cavernosum. The direct revascularization of the corpus cavernosum, a technique developed by Michal in 1973 [2] which now has an historic value, was followed by operations that have become continually more sophisticated and complex, with the aim of recreating a normal hemodynamic situation. Microsurgical techniques made possible the anastomosis between the inferior epigastric artery and the dorsal artery of the penis [3]. However, anatomic studies that have followed appear to negate the existence of an anastomotic network between the dorsal arteries of the penis and the arteries of the cavernosal body, the real factors responsible for the engorgement of the corpus cavernosum and the erectile deficiency.

Subsequently, alternate techniques such as the "upstream" (against the current) anastomoses between the inferior epigastric vessels and the dorsal artery of the penis [4] were developed; the inversion of the flow permits a reverse passage of blood towards the cavernosal artery (Fig. 1). In 1982 Crespo [5] proposed an operation based on a direct anastomosis between the epigastric artery and the cavernosal artery. This procedure was quickly abandoned due to the difficulty in finding this miniscule vessel inside the cavernosal tissue. The continual experience gained from this type of surgery and the analysis of the results obtained led to the development of new concepts and to the birth of alternate surgical procedures. In 1986 Hauri [6] proposed a new type of operation based on the anastomosis between the epigastric artery, deep dorsal vein, and dorsal artery. This was based on his observation that in vascular surgery of the peripheral circulation the creation of an arterial-venous fistula at the point where the arteriolo-arteriolare anastomosis takes place, reduces the risk of thrombosis by improving the blood flow. A variation of this technique uses an anastomosis between the epigastric artery, dorsal penile vein, and corpus cavernosum (Fig. 2) [7]. If occlusion or extremely small caliber of the vessel makes it impossible to perform an anastomosis

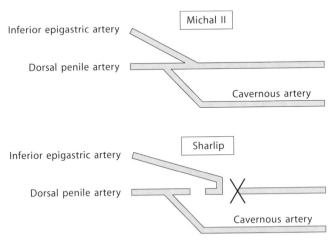

Fig. 1. Techniques of penile arterial revascularization according to Michal and Sharlip

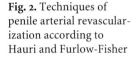

Fig. 2. Techniques of penile arterial revascularization according to Hauri and Furlow-Fisher

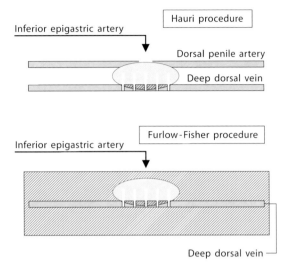

with the principal arterial trunks of the penis (dorsal and cavernosal arteries), Virag has proposed techniques for anastomosis of the epigastric artery or a saphenous graft between femoral artery and the dorsal penile vein (Fig. 3).

However, these techniques, though well supported by rigorous hemodynamic principles, have seen few innovations, and in practice they have not brought about substantial improvements in final results. Follow-up arteriographic examinations show eventual occlusion of the fistula due to the presence of turbulence, with an accompanying reduction in the velocity of the blood flow. The lack of positive results have led many to believe that future improvements in surgery to cure erectile dysfunction require not only a better understanding of the erectile mechanism but also a more careful selection of patients. Only the stenosis or the segmentary occlusion of the functional arteries of the penis can be treated by a revascularization operative procedure.

Those who must be excluded as candidates include patients with associated pathologies, those with diffuse atherosclerosis which has spread to other areas, and those showing other risk factors concomitant with erectile deficit. Diabetics, hypertensive patients, heavy cigarette smokers, and men over 50 years old are also not ideal candidates for revascularization of the penis. Prosthetic therapy is undoubtedly preferred in these cases. This modern approach to the surgical therapy of erectile dysfunction has

Fig. 3. Techniques of penile arterial revascularization according to Virag

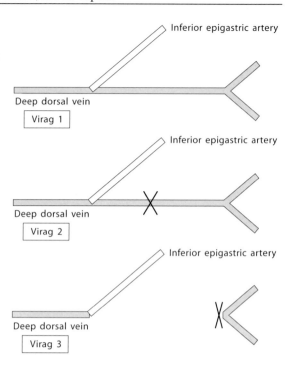

completely modified the indications for functional reconstructive surgery of an erection, and it is the only therapy capable of providing satisfying results. The success rate is about 75% in cases selected according to the above criteria, and about 25% in subjects in whom erectile dysfunction is associated with vascular diseases resulting from diffuse atherosclerosis. The best results are obtained in patients in whom the vascular lesion is due to trauma of the minor pelvis. In conclusion, the real progress in long-term results does not lie in a particular microsurgical technique but in the careful selection of the patients, rendered possible by the sophisticated diagnostic techniques that are continually being improved.

Surgical Treatment of Erectile Dysfunction
due to Failure of the Veno-occlusive Mechanisms

The role of the penile venous system in the mechanism of an erection is still not completely known. The venous drainage in the penis is accomplished by numerous systems:

- The superficial dorsal vein, a derivative of the external pudendal vein, is situated between the skin and the fascia of Buck, at the point where the venous branches from the foreskin and the penile shaft join. These vessels are a tributary of the great saphenous vein.
- The deep dorsal vein (DDV), which runs from the two cavernosal bodies in the space between the fascia of Buck and the tunica albuginea, receives vessels originating from the glans penis and the corpus spongiosum from the urethra and in turn derives from the periprostatic plexus of Santorini. This network maintains multiple connections with the superficial venous system.
- The bulbourethral veins are an auxiliary system that drains the corpus spongiosum.
- The cavernosal veins, situated deep in the tunica albuginea, is the main drainage system for the corpus cavernosum. They drain into the vesicoprostatic plexus by means of four or five effluent branches which emerge in proximity to the crural root.
- The circumflex veins (perforating branches of the tunica albuginea) are distributed along the penile circumference and anastomizes with the deep venous system, and participate in the drainage of the corpus spongiosum.

The central physiological event of the erection is considered to be the relaxation of the smooth muscle component of the cavernosal tissue [8]. During the course of the erection this transforms the system of high resistance of the vascular lacunae into a low resistance vascular network. This increases arterial flow while a compression of the subalbuginea venulae reduces the venous flow. These two events cause the entrapment of blood inside the corpus cavernosum, producing the penile tumescence and rigidity which are essential for penetration. Thus the venous component in the physiology of the erection has a substantially passive role, despite the fact that some experts have reported the presence of α-receptors on the inside of the vein walls [9, 10]. Belief in the active role of the penile venous system, which was widespread in the 1980s, probably explains the high number of failures reported for the various surgical techniques used in cases of venous leakage.

Diagnoses suggested by data collected from the patient's history of venous leakage, characterized by an insufficient degree of rigidity for penetration, have been improved on the basis of radiological (cavernosography) and instrumental (cavernosometry) examinations, techniques that are continually being revised. Dynamic cavernosography is influenced by numerous variables, particularly the patient's individual response to vasoactive drugs, tropisms of the corpus cavernosal tissue, and the sympathetic tone, which depends upon the emotional state of the patient. The radiological demonstration of venous leakage is a limited diagnostic tool. In addition to being an extremely invasive examination with potentially severe side effects (e.g., contrast solution reactions, fibrosis of the corpus cavernosum) it has low sensitivity and is associated with a high rate of false positives. Even when the site at which the venous leakage takes place can be visualized in the contrast solution, it is of limited therapeutic value; the surgical procedure is limited to the tying off and the eventual excision of the DDV, or in the case of a massive leakage at the crura it can be wrapped. The same factors that influence the results of dynamic cavernosography are the basis for the errors in interpretating the results of cavernosometry, which does not consider arterial flow to the penis or organic or functional alterations in the cavernosal tissue.

The picture of "venous leakage" presented by dynamic cavernosography and cavernosometry in patients suffering primarily from inability to maintain an erection is essentially due to an underlying alteration in one or more erectile mechanisms of an organic or functional origin, classifiable as an insufficiency in veno-occlusive function. The surgical approach to these cases can vary. Some studies have involved a simple tying off of the DDV [11, 12], others the tying off and excising only the DDV [13, 21], and in others in addition to tying off the cavernosal veins [22] the crura [23–26] was also tied and spongiosolysis [27] tried. In some series a considerable number of circumflex veins were tied off. It is therefore easy to understand why the surgical therapy of veno-occlusive insufficiency, despite being a relatively simple procedure to perform, is accompanied by a high incidence of failures [11, 13–16, 18, 21, 25, 27]. In the series with high success rates (70%–75%) [12, 17, 19, 20, 22–24] follow-up was carried out too soon in order to arrive at a definitive conclusion. In our experience [26] only two patients (28%) suffering from veno-occlusive dysfunction have achieved optimal recovery of erectile function (rigidity and duration), with a corresponding improvement in cavernosometric parameters, 12 months after the operation. Some patients recorded only a slight improvement in the number of nocturnal erections, along with a corresponding reduction in the maintenance flow during the course of cavernosometry, without recovering a satisfactory sexual life. In 44% of the cases there was no significant improvement following the surgery.

Failure of the surgery is undoubtedly not due to a defect in the procedure itself; rather, the events leading to the diagnosis of venous leakage and the rationale behind all the procedures involving venous surgery must be incriminated. Certain arguments should be pointed out: (a) no operation can resolve the underlying pathology of the corpus cavernosum; (b) the surgical procedure is not capable of closing all of the venous branches, particularly the cavernosal veins, which is hard to reach and is often involved in the mechanism of "leakage"; (c) with time collateral pathways for the venous drainage develop, which explains the high number of relapses. Surgical therapy for "venous leakage" is limited today to creating a temporary obstacle for the blood flow. Analysis of the "veno-occlusive dysfunction" syndrome and the basis for the strategy of an appropriate therapy require additional studies of the morphological, biochemical, and functional aspects of the cavernosal tissue.

Prosthetic Therapy

The ideal candidate for a penile prosthesis is a patient suffering from erectile deficiency of an organic nature, in a condition that has been stable for a relatively long period of time, and unable to be treated with presently available medical therapy. Obviously the candidate must still have sexual desire (libido), sensitivity of the penis, orgasm, and ejaculation. There are several types of prostheses available today, and the choice among them is based upon a series of technical and psychological considerations (Table 1). For this reason an interview with the patient and

Table 1. Classification of penile prostheses

Semi-rigid	Malleable	Hydraulic	Mechanical
Small Carrion (Mentor) Flexi-Rod (Surgitek) Duraphase (Dacomed) Subrini	AM 600 (AMS-Pfizer) Jonas (Bard) Mentor Malleable (Mentor)	Self-Contained Flexi-Flate (Surgitek) Hydroflex (AMS-Pfizer) Dynaflex (AMS-Pfizer) *Two-component* Uniflate 1000 (Surgitek) Mentor Mark II (Mentor) *Three-component* AMS 700 CX (AMS-Pfizer) Mentor Alfa-1 (Mentor)	Omniphase (Dacomed)

his partner is indispensable since it provides the physician an understanding of the motivation for the choice and the intellectual condition of the subject. The cost of the various prostheses must also be considered because this can vary considerably, as well as the costs of the implantation (operating room, surgical team, hospital stay, etc.) and those involved in complications that can arise. Important factors in this decision are also the experience of the surgeon and his personal preference.

Semirigid and Malleable Prostheses

Semirigid prostheses are composed of two silicone cylinders inserted inside the corpus cavernosum by means of a perineal, penoscrotal, or infrapubic incision. It differs from the rigid prosthesis in that these models have a hinge positioned at the point where the anterior two-thirds meets the posterior two-thirds of the cylinder. This last portion is inserted inside the crura and represents the fixed portion of the prosthesis.

To activate the prosthesis, the cylinders are manually turned up, while at "rest" they are positioned laterally or turned down. The malleable prosthesis has a metallic support that permits it to be bent or extended according to the patient's necessity. This type of prosthesis is available in different lengths and diameters. The large variety is justified by the fact that prior to surgery it is very difficult to determine the length of the corpus cavernosum. The cost is very reasonable, and the procedure relatively simple. We do not wish to oversimplify this procedure because numerous problems do exist which can arise from the implantation of this type of prosthesis. The models that have an internal metal support, such as the Jonas, are subject to frequent mechanical problems due to the failure of the internal cable [28]. The constant rigidity of the penis can produce considerable esthetic problems and often produces a compressive ischemic condition which can result in tissue necrosis and expulsion of the cylinder. During sexual intercourse there exists the risk of breaking through to the crura or the glandular apex of the corpus cavernosum. These types of implants are reserved for elderly candidates or those with severe problems in the area where the implantation is normally placed.

Mechanical Prostheses

Mechanical prostheses deserve mention only for the originality of their construction. They are made of cylinders composed of articulated metallic rings. On the inside of the cylinder there is a steel cable suspended by two springs that put tension upon the various components when the prosthesis is activated. This mechanism makes a considerable amount of noise when it is activated, and this is worsened by the fact that there is a high complication rate due to failure of the metal cable.

Hydraulic Prostheses

Comparing a semi-rigid or malleable prosthesis to an hydraulically activated mono-, bi-, or tricomponent prosthesis clearly demonstrates the progress that has been made in recent years. Despite all the advances that have been made in this field, however, today there still does not exist an ideal prosthetic device capable of satisfying every type of patient, regardless of age, underlying pathology, and individual expectations. The types of hydraulic prostheses available today are outlined above. Their construction and the way in which they function appear obsolete [29–31]. Here we discuss the principal characteristics of the various models and the major advantages or disadvantages of their implantation.

The triple component models are undoubtedly the most advanced types from a technical and functional-esthetic standpoint. This type of prosthesis permits an almost complete state of flaccidity and one of rigidity; it is also possible to substantially expand the diameters of the cylinders thanks to the abundant supply of liquid in the reservoir. The Ultrex model AMS is even able to increase in length as well as circumference thanks to the spatial arrangement (spiral) of the molecules of silicone. Naturally their implantation is more complex and not always possible, especially in patients who have undergone abdominal-pelvic surgery or radiation treatment for neoplasms in the pelvis. In addition, it is quite expensive. The single-component models are relatively easy to implant, and the cost is more reasonable. However, with these the subject never reaches a complete state of flaccidity or rigidity and considering the reduced amount of fluid contained in the cylinders, it is also not possible to obtain a concomitant increase in the diameter of the penis. The most recent models such as the Dynaflex are able to increase slightly the diameter of the penis thanks, again, to the disposition of the fibers of silicone. A number of models no longer on the market had functional problems such as the "spontaneous" deflation of the prosthesis following microtrauma resulting from the sexual intercourse.

These inconveniences in some cases required the removal and substitution of the devices. The bicomponent models appear to offer three undisputable advantages: low cost, good esthetic and functional results, and ease of implantation. However, the valve-controlled reservoir positioned in an intrascrotal position is very cumbersome, and the reduced quantity of liquid contained in the system permits only a modest increase in the diameter of the cylinders, certainly in no way comparable to the capacity of the tricomponent prosthesis.

Soft Prostheses

A very recent proposal has a new type of prosthesis made of "soft" silicone. This prosthesis is implanted inside the corpus cavernosum, not to increase the rigidity of the shaft but to reduce the "dead" spaces in the cavernosal tissue. This makes a smaller quantity of blood necessary to produce an erection of the penis. These prostheses take advantage of the residual erection of the subject and are indicated for patients suffering from an erection deficiency of a psychogenic origin and who do not respond to medical therapy, or whose vascular erectile dysfunction results from venous "leakage".

Surgical Techniques

Penile prostheses can be inserted into the corpus cavernosum by the following routes: perineal, mediopenile, penoscrotal, transscrotal, infrapubic, and subcoronal. There is no general rule, and the choice of surgical approach is left to the surgeon on the basis of his experience and the type of prosthesis to be implanted.

From our personal experience, we prefer to position the prosthesis using the transscrotal approach, making a small transverse incision or using the Scott autostatic retractor, which permits an excellent bilateral view of the corpus cavernosa. In difficult cases such as reoperations, positioning an alloplastic patch for induratio penis plastica or fibrosis of the corpus cavernosi, it is possible to extend the incision, using the same approach with no difficulty. The subcoronal entry is indicated for positioning rigid or mechanical prostheses. In conclusion, of the possible entries available to the surgeon he must be very careful not to damage the urethra when using the ventral approach, or the neurovascular fascia when making a dorsal entry, as damaging any of these structures can markedly compromise the sensitivity of the glans. The incision, made with an electric scalpel, which limits the bleeding, must not be greater that 2–3 cm. Before dilating the corpus cavernosum a pair of Metzenbaum scissors is inserted into them through the incision. This is very important because it serves to create the correct pathway for the subsequent dilation, sectioning any fibrous offshoots that are still present, particularly in patients with certain pathologies (e.g., induratio penis plastica resulting from intracavernosal injections of vasoactive drugs). The corpus cavernosum must be dilated very carefully, trying to arrive at the distal and proximal extremities without perforating the albuginea.

For this part of the procedure we find it extremely helpful to use a Dilamezin set or, as a possible alternative, a set of Brooks, which by their form permit excellent maneuverability and a uniform dilation of the corpus cavernosal, which we have verified in a study on cadavers. Measuring the length of the corpus cavernosum is very important, for insertion of a prosthesis of the correct dimensions is a fundamental requirement for a successful outcome of the operation. A prosthesis that is too long can perforate the corpus cavernosum during sexual activity and provoke perineal pain, and one that is too short can cause the phenomenon known as Concorde deformity and render penetration impossible. Some models of hydraulic prostheses include extensions at the proximal extremity of the cylinder (rear tip extender) whose purpose is to obtain a length very similar to that of the corpus cavernosum. In other types of prostheses these extensions are substituted by a segment made from silicone which can be cut off with a pair of scissors or sharp blade. In general, it is a good rule to place the longest cylinder possible, using the shortest extension. Careful attention must be made when closing the incision, especially if a hydraulic prosthesis is implanted, not to penetrate the cylinder with the suture, which would cause irreparable damage. To prevent this from happening disposable little "spatules" are provided which protect the cylinder when closing the incision. With prosthesis composed of two or three components it is important to avoid bending the tubes by positioning as many layers as possible between the prosthesis and the cutaneous barrier.

Placing the multicomponent prostheses requires some more steps in positioning the pump and the reservoir than does the monocomponent device. The pump must be placed in the scrotum, a position which is convenient for the subject, relatively immobile, and able to be grasped by one hand. Therefore we consider the subdartoica portion of the scrotum the ideal location for its emplacement. The reservoir can be placed in the perivesicular space or internally in the peritoneal cavity. Our experience shows the latter site to be the most suitable, due principally to the fact that it is possible to use a larger capacity reservoir, such as the AMS 700

Ultrex (100 cm³), thereby providing a maximum level of filling and rigidity to the cylinders.

In addition, there is no risk of fibrotic trapping of the reservoir. This can cause problems in the future, such as involuntary autoactivation of the prosthesis. Therefore during the initial postoperative period the reservoir is left only partially filled, not needing to create a space in the new implantation site. Consequently, the cylinders, when completely filled with liquid, produce a hemostatic compression of the corpus cavernosum and prevent complications such as edema and bleeding. The positioning in the perivesicular site can also be used with a small-volume reservoir (65 cm³) or when it is intended to use the same transscrotal access to insert the reservoir, passing through the subcutaneous inguinal orifice and opening the transversalis fascia with the aid of a pair of scissors. Instruments have been purposely created for this procedure, permitting it to be performed with extreme ease and without the risk of damaging surrounding structures, such as the inferior epigastric vessels. Whenever this method is chosen for inserting the reservoir it is good practice to insert a catheter to avoid damaging the bladder.

Complications

One of the major problems encountered when implanting penile prostheses is that of controlling infections [31, 32]. For this reason particular precautions must be taken both before and during the operation. The candidate for the prosthetic implant must have no concomitant urinary infections; if he does, he must be treated immediately with an appropriate antibiotic. He must also have no cutaneous infections in or around the genital area. The patient must be shaved and prepared either in the operating room immediately prior to insertion of the prosthesis or in the ward a few hours prior to the surgery. In either case it is important to be very careful and avoid cutaneous lacerations that could be a source of bacterial contamination (sterile razor, gloves, and antiseptic prep solution).

Two days before surgery the patient is instructed to wash the perineal area with an iodized solution. On the morning of the operation he is treated prophylactically with antibiotics (gentamycin and vancomycin) to avoid staphylococcal infections and gram-negative urinary pathogens [33]. The antibiotic therapy is continued for at least 7 days after the operation. A mildly compressing medication is applied to the penis, and a urinary catheter K-30 is inserted for 24 h. The patient can resume sexual activity 4 weeks after the operation.

Conclusion

In conclusion, the operations for inserting prostheses are in themselves simple techniques to which one can resort, without any hesitation, when there is no alternative of less invasive therapy. Depending on the type of prosthesis used, this surgery offers a greater than a 95% chance of success.

Tricomponent prostheses undoubtedly offer better esthetic and functional results. The placement of these devices requires somewhat more attention and a minimum of experience in prosthetic surgery. These are particularly indicated in patients who have a penis of acceptable dimensions and have not undergone pelvic-abdominal surgery or, even worse, radiotherapy of the minor pelvis. Nevertheless even in patients who have undergone prior surgery in the lower abdominal region, it is possible to place the reservoir in an intraperitoneal position. It is very important in each case to discuss and explain to the patient the various prosthetic models that are available and the advantages and disadvantages of each. Even in this type of surgery we believe that the success of the operation depends mainly on the decisions that must be made after a complete andrological screening and after a careful consideration of the actual expectations of the patient.

References

1. Leriche R, Morel A (1948) The syndrome of thrombotic obliteration of the aortic bifurcation. Ann Surg 127:193
2. Michal V, Kramar R, Pospical J, Hejal L (1973) Direct arterial anastomosis on corpora cavernosa penis in therapy of erectile impotence. Rozhl Chir 52:587-590
3. Michal V, Kramar R, Pospical J et al (1980) Vascular surgery in the treatment of impotence: its present possibilities and prospects. Czech Med 3:213-217
4. Sharlip ID (1984) Retrograde revascularization of the deep penile artery for arteriogenic erectile dysfunction. J Urol 131:513 (232 A)
5. Crespo E, Soltanik E, Bove D, Farrell G (1982) Treatment of vasculogenic sexual impotence by revascularizing cavernous and/or dorsal arteries using microvascular techniques. Urology 20:271-275
6. Hauri D (1986) A new operative technique in vasculogenic erectile impotence. World J Urol 4:237
7. Furlow WL, Fisher J, Knoll LD (1988) Penile revascularization: experience with deep dorsal vein arterialization – the Furlow-Fisher modification – with 27 patients. In: Proceedings of the Sixth Biennal Symposium for Corpus Cavernosum Revascularization & Third Biennal World Meeting on Impotence. International Society for Impotence Research (ISIR), Boston, p139
8. Saenz de Tejada I, Goldstein I, Krane RJ (1988) Local control of penile erection. Nerves, smooth muscle , and endothelium. Urol Clin North Am 15:9
9. Fontaine J, Schulmann CC, Wespes E (1987) Postjunctional alpha-1- and alpha-2-like activity in human isolated deep dorsal vein of the penis. Br J Pharmacol 89:493
10. Kirkeby HJ, Fordan A, Sorensen S, Anderson KE (1989) Alpha-adrenoreceptor function in isolated penile circumflex veins from potent and impotent patients. J Urol 142:1369-1371
11. Austoni E, Bellorofonte C, Mantovani F (1987) Improved results with intracavernous drug infusion following new surgical techniques for vasculogenic impotence. World J Urol 5:182-189
12. Wespes E, Schulman CC (1985) Venous leakage: surgical treatment of a curable cause of impotence. J Urol 133: 796-798
13. Wespes E (1991) Diagnostic and surgical approach to impotent patients with cavernous leakage. In: Jonas U, Thon WF, Stief CG (eds) Erectile dysfunction. Springer, Berlin Heidelberg New York, pp282-290
14. Parrott LH, Sholes AH, Rice JC, Lewis RW, Kerstein MD (1989) Penile vein dissection: a study of its long-term efficacy in impotence. World J Urol 7:169-172
15. Lewis RW (1988) Venous surgery for impotence. Urol Clin North Am 15(1):115-121
16. Lewis RW, Puyau FA, Bell DP (1987) Another surgical approach for vasculogenic impotence. J Urol 136:1210-1212
17. Bennet AH, Rivard DJ, Blanc RP, Moran M (1986) Reconstructive surgery for vasculogenic impotence. J Urol 136: 599

18. Lunglmayr G, Nachtingall M, Gindl K (1988) Long-term results of deep dorsal penile vein transection in venous impotence. Eur Urol 15: 209-212
19. Williams G, Mulcahy MJ, Hartnell G, Kiely E (1988) Diagnosis and treatment of venous leakage: a curable cause of impotence. Br J Urol 61: 151-155
20. Treiber U, Gilbert P (1989) Venous surgery in erectile dysfunction: a critical report on 116 patients. Urology 34: 22-27
21. Buvat G, Lemaire A, Buvat-Herbaut M, Dehaene J, Marcolin G, Desmons F (1980) Impuissances avec fuite veneuse. Ann Urol (Paris) 20 (5):323-330
22. Lue TF (1989) Penile venous surgery. Urol Clin North Am 16:607-611
23. Puech-Leao Reis JMSM, Glina S, Reichelt AC (1987) Leakage through the crural edge of corpus cavernosum. Eur Urol 13:163-165
24. Bar Moshe O, Vandendris M (1988) Treatment of impotence due to perineal venous leakage by ligation of crura penis. J Urol 139: 1217-1219
25. Glina S, Leao PP, Marcondes Dos Reis JM, Reichelt AC, Chao S (1993) Surgical exclusion of the crural ending of the corpora cavernosa: late results. Eur Urol
26. Carmignani G, Ciampalini S, De Stefani S, Simonato A, Capone M (1991) Valutazione obiettivostrumentale nelle insufficienze veno-occlusive sottoposte a legatura della crura. Atti VII Congress Società Italiana Andrologia, Monduzzi, Milan, pp323-326
27. Gilbert P, Stief C (1987) Spongiosolysis: a new surgical treatment of impotence caused by distal venous leakage. JUrol 138:784-786
28. Jonas U (1983) 5-years' experience with the silicone-silver penile prothesis: improvements and new developments. World J Urol 1:251
29. American Medical System Inc. A report of the clinical evaluation of the 700 Ultrex TM penile prothesis. AMS publication 00926
30. Mentor Corp. Mark II inflatable prothesis. Surgical protocol. Mentor Corporation
31. Thomalla JV, Thompson ST, Rowland RG, Mulcahy JJ (1987) Infectious complications of penile prosthetic implants. J Urol 138:65
32. Carson CC, Robertson CN (1988) Late hematogenous infection of penile prostheses. J Urol 139-150
33. Maffezzini M, De Stefani S, Ciampalini S, Bianco S, Capone M, Simonato A, Carmignani G (1991) La profilassi antibiotica nella terapia protesica dei genitali esterni. Acta Urol Ital 5:333-335

Peyronie's Disease
and Vasculogenic Erectile Dysfunction

J.A. VALE

Introduction

Peyronie's disease, or induratio penis plastica, is penile curvature during erection which develops as a result of fibrosis within the tunica albuginea (the tough elastic capsule of the corpus cavernosum). Although it was first described in 1561 by Fallopius, it was popularised by and named after Francois de la Peyronie [1], surgeon to Louis XV of France. It is not uncommon within the general population, with a prevalence rate of about 388/100 000 population and an average age-adjusted incidence of 25.7/100 000 men per year [2].

The pathology of Peyronie's is well known, with an area of fibrosis/scar tissue and a reduction in the proportion of elastin fibres in the tunica albuginea [3] causing penile curvature due to failure of normal penile lengthening on the affected side. However, the aetiology remains unresolved. The most widely accepted theory is that it results from mild trauma leading to bleeding within the tunica albuginea [4]. As the resulting clot is resorbed, fibrin remains in the injured tissue, and there is activation of fibroblasts and inflammatory mediators within the site as part of the normal process of repair. It is this phase that may be associated with pain in some patients. The entire process of fibrin deposition and attempts at repair takes about 12–18 months, consistent with the period over which the penile curvature tends to stabilise.

The trauma theory for the development of scar tissue fits with many of the features of Peyronie's disease, including a history of mild sexual trauma in the weeks prior to onset in some patients. However, it is hard to prove such a mechanism as all evidence is anecdotal and retrospective, and there are some features of the disease that are hard to explain on this basis. Firstly, changes in the structure and organisation of collagen fibres have been noted in the contralateral "unaffected" tunica albuginea of patients with Peyronie's disease [5]. Secondly, there is an association between Peyronie's disease and other fibromatous disorders, including Dupuytren's contracture [6], and an association has been shown between these conditions and chronic barbiturate administration [7]. Thirdly, the HLA class II antigens HLA-DR3 and HLA-DQw2 are significantly more common amongst men with Peyronie's disease than in the general population [8].

The above facts all suggest that there may be systemic factors in the development of Peyronie's disease, especially as HLA-DR3 and DQw2 are typically associated with organospecific autoimmune disorders. Patients with Peyronie's have higher levels of antibodies to tropoelastin and alpha-elastin than age-matched controls [9], and it is possible that auto-immune mechanisms may have a role in the development of this condition.

Peyronie's Disease and Erectile Dysfunction

Amongst men presenting with erectile dysfunction, Peyronie's disease may be present in up to 20% [10] and is frequently unsuspected; the diagnosis may only be made at the time of colour Doppler imaging (CDI) of the vasculature. Of those patients who present with Peyronie's disease about 30%–40% will have erectile dysfunction [3, 11]. Some authors have suggested that the association is not one of cause and effect [11], but given the frequency of the association and the importance of the tunica albuginea in erectile mechanisms it seems likely that they are causally related. Studies in patients with Peyronie's disease and erectile dysfunction have shown evidence of penile arterial pathology in 36% and apparent veno-occlusive failure in 18%–59% [10, 12]. In one series [10] the plaque was actually observed to distort the vessels in 20% of patients, and it is this spread of fibrosis into the corpus cavernosum that probably causes arterial stenosis. Development of veno-occlusive failure is more difficult to explain, but there are two possible mechanisms. Firstly, fibrosis causes a change in the flexibility of the tunica albuginea, making it relatively stiff. During a normal erection the emissary veins passing through the tunica are occluded by the tension within the tunical wall.

Obviously, if the tunica is rigid and inelastic, this passive mechanism may fail. Secondly, if Peyronie's disease develops as a result of trauma to the erect penis, as has been suggested, the trauma may also precipitate haemodynamic pathology. Penson et al. [13] performed pharmacocavernosometry/cavernosography in 19 patients with erectile dysfunction and a definite history of blunt trauma to the erect penis and found that 79% had evidence of site-specific venous leakage. In a biomechanical model they showed that sudden penile loading could produce intracavernosal pressures exceeding 900 mmHg; this abrupt rise in pressure could have a damaging effect on venous and tunical tissue alike. Thus venous leakage might develop as the result of a single acute event, whilst arterial stenosis is likely to develop more insidiously as fibrosis spreads from the tunica to the corpus cavernosum.

In summary, erectile failure occurring in association with Peyronie's disease may be arteriogenic, venogenic, or mixed vascular. In addition, however, there may be no apparent vascular pathology on CDI, suggesting a psychogenic picture; this is more common in patients with a uniform loss of erection than in those complaining of distal flaccidity [14]. The accurate assessment of patients prior to surgery for Peyronie's disease is thus very important; the only operative procedure that reliably improves vasculogenic erectile dysfunction is the insertion of a penile prosthesis.

Clinical Features

Peyronie's disease is most common in middle-aged men who are sexually active; it is relatively unusual in young men. This may be due to changes in the elasticity of the tunical tissue with ageing. The tunical tissue in young men is able to flex in response to lateral forces, whilst in the middle-aged man it is less elastic and tends to tear. Peyronie's disease is relatively uncommon in the elderly, presumably because intercourse is more restrained and perhaps less frequent.

The majority of patients present with a history of penile curvature, with difficult or impossible intercourse in 40% [15]. About a third of patients complain of penile pain during erection [15] and may present with a painful lump; these patients are probably relatively early in the evolution of their plaque, with a marked inflammatory reaction. As the plaque stabilises, the pain usually diminishes.

It is essential to take a careful sexual history during the patient's first consultation, with particular emphasis on erectile function. Examination should include inspection and palpation of the penile shaft to define the extent of a plaque, and the penis should be examined during an erection. This is best accomplished by administering an intracavernosal injection of papaverine or prostaglandin E_1, as this also demonstrates any associated failure of rigidity. Some clinicians rely upon the patient to take a polaroid photograph, but this may permit flaccidity distal to a plaque to go unnoticed.

A number of imaging modalities have been recommended for the assessment of Peyronie's disease, including high-resolution ultrasound, computed tomography, magnetic resonance imaging with or without gadolinium, and colour Doppler ultrasound. High-resolution ultrasound and computed tomography are effective methods of visualising Peyronie's plaques [16, 17], but they provide only anatomical information and in the presence of a palpable plaque have no diagnostic role in my opinion. Magnetic resonance imaging also provides details of the extent of plaque tissue, but when gadolinium is given, it also provides information about active inflammation if there is enhancement of the fibrous tissue [18] (Fig. 1). This may be useful in monitoring plaque evolution and per-

Fig. 1. Penile magnetic resonance image with gadolinium

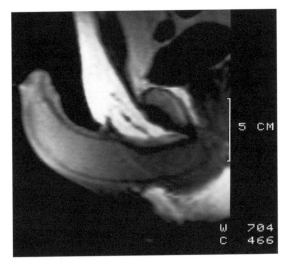

haps planning any surgical intervention. However, once again, it is unlikely that magnetic resonance imaging will have a role in the routine
evaluation of the Peyronie's patient. CDI is without doubt the investigation of choice if imaging is indicated, especially if there is a history of any
erectile failure. It can be used to assess vascular function as well as defining plaque anatomy (Fig. 2).

Treatment of Peyronie's Disease

There are really three treatment options in Peyronie's disease: medical
therapy, surgical correction of angulation, and no treatment at all. If the
patient is pain free and able to have intercourse without difficulty, clearly
no treatment is necessary. Most patients are satisfied with this once the
benign and self-limiting nature of Peyronie's disease has been explained

Fig. 2. Penile echo colour
Doppler image. It is
possible to appreciate the
alteration of the cavernosal tissue, the distortion
of the cavernosal artery
and some areas of fibrosis
(in green)

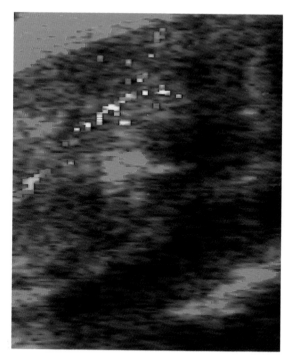

to them. I usually advise the patient to return in the future if the curvature increases, or erectile function deteriorates.

Medical Therapies

If the patient complains of pain from the site of the plaque, this suggests that the condition is still evolving. It is this group of men who might benefit from medical treatment, and a number of treatment options are available. However, most have not been subjected to a rigorous randomised controlled trial, and the end-point is usually highly subjective, such as perceived improvement in curvature or reduced difficulty in having intercourse. Perhaps the best known therapy is potassium aminobenzoate, which is believed to have antifibroblastic activity. It is taken as an oral dose of 12 g per day, and up to one third of patients are unable to tolerate it due to gastrointestinal side effects. Some studies have cast doubt on its efficacy [19]. Vitamin E has also been recommended in the treatment of Peyronie's disease, at a dose of 600–800 mg per day in divided doses, and this may produce improvement or at least prevent progression in two thirds of patients [20]. Once again, the evidence is highly subjective, but it is without side effect, and it may be worthwhile in patients presenting with a painful plaque and an evolving curvature. These patients are not candidates for surgery until their disease has stabilised. Tamoxifen at 40 mg per day has also been used in these circumstances, and produced a reduction in penile pain in 80% of patients. It was less effective in correcting penile deformity, with only a third of patients reporting any change [21].

Other more aggressive medical therapies have also been tried, including intralesional injections of steroids, verapamil [22] collagenase [23] and radiotherapy [24]. The latter, administered at a dose of 9–16 Gy using orthovoltage techniques, is very effective at producing a rapid resolution of pain but has little effect on curvature or erectile dysfunction.

In general in medicine there is an inverse relationship between the number of treatments for a condition and their efficacy. This certainly seems to be true for Peyronie's disease, and if I had to propose a rational approach for the treatment of the patient with a painful plaque I would start with vitamin E, proceed to potassium aminobenzoate or tamoxifen, and reserve orthovoltage radiotherapy for patients with refractory pain not responding to these measures. I do not believe that medical therapy has any role in patients with painless established deformity.

Surgery

Surgery is appropriate only when the plaque has stabilised, and the deformity is no longer progressing; there is no point correcting 30° of angulation only to find that 6 months later a further 10° of deformity has developed. Stabilisation of the plaque usually corresponds to the cessation of pain in those patients in whom it was a feature, and I usually wait a further 6 months to be certain that the deformity is static.

In general, patients with an upward bend of less than 45° can usually manage satisfactory intercourse, whilst 30° is the critical angle for downward or lateral angulation. Some patients deny the feasibility of intercourse with even very mild degrees of angulation because they are embarrassed by any degree of deformity. These patients represent a particular management problem.

Before undertaking any form of surgery it is mandatory to establish whether there is any degree of erectile failure. This may have a bearing on the surgical approach chosen, and in addition it is a useful baseline if the patient subsequently claims that surgery has reduced the quality of his erections. Intracavernosal injection with papaverine or prostaglandin E_1 is a satisfactory screening test, with CDI being reserved for those who fail to respond.

If the patient is normally potent, then surgical options include either excision of the plaque and a dermal inlay graft, or the rather simpler Nesbit operation. The disadvantage of the latter procedure is that it involves shortening the contralateral corpus cavernosum, leading to a degree of penile shortening overall. The degree of shortening is proportional to the degree of angulation that requires correction and may not be acceptable on a relatively small penis.

The Nesbit operation is performed via a circumcision-type incision with mobilisation of the penile shaft skin. An artificial erection is induced using a tourniquet and saline infusion, and the site of the plaque is identified; Buck's fascia is dissected off the contralateral corpus cavernosum at the opposite point on the penile circumference. If the plaque is on the ventral aspect of the penis, great care must be taken to mobilise the dorsal arteries and nerves within Buck's fascia dorsally before making any incisons in the tunica. If the plaque is on the dorsal aspect of the penis, the corpus spongiosum and contained urethra requires mobilisation before an ellipse of tunica is removed. An ellipse of tunica is then excised, its long axis lying transversely; care is taken not to damage the corpus cavernosal tissue at this stage. The defect is closed transversely using a slowly dissolving suture such as 3/0 polydiaoxanone. Occasionally it is necessary to excise more than one ellipse in order to achieve the desired degree of straightening, and at the end of the procedure it is necessary to produce a further artificial erection to ensure that the penis is straight. Buck's fascia is closed over the corporotomy site, and the circumcision incision is closed using interrupted catgut or 4/0 undied vicryl or dexon. Patients are given desipramine 75 mg daily in divided doses for 2 weeks to prevent erections and are advised to avoid intercourse for a month.

Some surgeons have modified the Nesbit operation and instead of excising an ellipse of tunica to achieve shortening the corpus is plicated using a non-absorbable suture such as 2/0 prolene. The results are very similar, and in a recent outcome study 82% of patients were able to have normal intercourse after penile plication for Peyronie's disease as compared to only 8% pre-operatively [25]. In the same study 42% of partners complained of discomfort prior to surgery, whereas this number had reduced to 4% post-operatively.

If there is concern about penile shortening, an alternative strategy is to excise the plaque itself and replace the diseased area with a patch/graft of some kind. Various types of patch have been used including artificial materials such as Dacron or Gore-Tex, but these have proved unsatisfactory due to their lack of elasticicty and a tendency to cause local inflammation and perhaps fibrosis. A graft from the dermal layer of non-hair bearing skin appears to be most suitable [20], and the graft is usually taken from the flank just above the iliac crest. The basic approach for the operation is similar to that for a Nesbit operation, a circumcision incision being suitable in most cases and the dorsal arteries and nerves or the corpus spongiosum being mobilised as necessary. An artificial erection is induced, and the plaque is fully identified and excised carefully avoiding darmage to the underlying cavernosal tissue.

The size of the resulting defect is carefully measured, and an appropriate area of skin is chosen and marked out. The epidermis is removed from the underlying dermis with a sharp scalpel, and then the dermis is excised as a free graft. The graft is sutured to the tunical edge of the defect using a continuous water-tight layer of 5/0 polydiaoxanone. An artificial erection is produced to ensure that the penis is straight and the graft is water-tight. Buck's fascia is re-approximated over the corporal tissue and lightly tacked with 3/0 vicryl, and the circumcision incision is closed. The graft donor site is closed by mobilising the skin edges to prevent puckering, and then a subcuticular suture is used.

Results of dermal inlay surgery have been satisfactory, with an overall patient satisfaction rate of 70%, and 53% of patients who were previously unable to have intercourse were able to resume intercourse after surgery [26]. The most frequent complication of this surgery is recurrent curvature due to graft retraction; this occurred in 35% of patients in one series [27]. To minimise the risk of this, a dermal graft approximately 30% larger than the corporotomy defect should be used, and patients should be encouraged to have erections as early as 2 weeks post-operatively to stretch the graft [4]. The second complication that has been reported after plaque excision and dermal graft surgery is a variable rate of erectile dysfunction in the range 12%–70% [26, 28]. This appears to represent veno-occlusive failure [29], presumably secondary to a disruption of the normal tunical passive venous occlusion mechanism. However, it has been suggested that the cause may be psychogenic in as many as 75% of patients with post-operative erectile dysfunction [30].

In patients with Peyronie's disease and erectile dysfunction the treatment of choice is the insertion of a penile prosthesis as there is little likelihood that correction of curvature will have any bearing on erectile function. Insertion of the prosthesis may be sufficient to cause straightening without any further surgical measures. However, in about half of patients it may be necessary to incise the plaque at the time of prosthesis insertion, and in exceptional circumstances plaque excision and an inlay graft may be required [31]. The use of penile prostheses has produced satisfactory results in general [31, 32], although a recent series has suggested that semi-rigid prostheses are associated with low patient and partner satisfaction rates of about 50% [33]. Inflatable prostheses are more satisfactory [34], and with recent improvements in reliability these are likely to become increasingly acceptable.

References

1. De la Peyronie F (1743) Sur quelques obstacles qui s'opposent a l'ejaculation naturelle de la semance. Mem Acad Chir 1:318
2. Lindsay MB, Schain DM, Grambsch P, Benson RC, Beard CM, Kurland LT (1991) The incidence of Peyronie's disease in Rochester, Minnesota 1950 through 1984. J Urol 146:1007–1009
3. Iacono F, Barra S, De Rosa G, Boscaino A, Lotti T (1993) Microstructural disorders of tunica albuginea in patients affected by Peyronie's disease with or without erectile dysfunction. J Urol 150:1806–1809
4. Devine CJ Jr, Jordan GH, Schlossberg SM (1992) Peyronie's disease. In: Walsh PC, Retik AB, Stamey TA, Vaughan ED Jr (eds) Campbell's urology. Saunders, Philadelphia, pp 3011–3022
5. Anafarta K, Beduk Y, Uluoglu O, Aydos K, Baltaci S (1994) The significance of histopathological changes of the normal tunica albuginea in Peyronie's disease. Int Urol Nephrol 26:71–77
6. Billig R, Baker R, Immergut M, Maxted W (1975) Peyronie's disease. Urology 6:409
7. Mattson RH, Cramer JA, McCutchen CB (1989) Barbiturate-related connective tissue disorders. Arch Intern Med 149:911–914
8. Rompel R, Mueller EG, Schroeder PI, Weidner W (1994) HLA antigens in Peyronie's disease. Urol Int 52:34–37
9. Stewart S, Malto M, Sandberg L, Colburn KK (1994) Increased levels of anti-elastin antibodies in patients with Peyronie's disease. J Urol 152:105–106
10. Amin Z, Patel U, Friedman EP, Vale JA, Kirby RS, Lees WR (1993) Colour Doppler and duplex assessment of Peyronie's disease in impotent men. Br J Radiol 66:398–402
11. Stecker JF, Devine CJ Jr (1984) Evaluation of erectile dysfunction in patients with Peyronie's disease. J Urol 132:680–681
12. Lopez JA, Jarow JP (1993) Penile vascular evaluation of men with Peyronie's disease. J Urol 149:53–55
13. Penson DF, Seftel AD, Krane RJ, Frohrib D, Goldstein I (1992) The haemodynamic pathophysiology of impotence following blunt trauma to the erect penis. J Urol 148:1171–1180
14. Ralph DJ, Hughes T, Lees WR, Pryor JP (1992) Pre-operative assessment of Peyronie's disease using colour Doppler sonography. Br J Urol 69:629–632
15. Wagenknecht LV, Meyer WH, Wiskemann A (1982) Value of various therapeutic procedures in penile induration. Urol Int 37:335–348
16. Balconi G, Angeli E, Nessi R, De-Flavilis L (1988) Ultrasonographic evaluation of Peyronie's disease. Urol Radiol 10:85–88
17. Rollandi GA, Tentarelli T, Vespier M (1985) Computed tomographic findings in Peyronie's disease. Urol Radiol 7:153–156
18. Helweg G, Judmaier W, Buchberger W, Wicke K, Oberhauser H, Knapp R, Ennemoser O, Zur-Nedden D (1992) Peyronie's disease: MR findings in 28 patients. Am J Roentgenol 158:1261–1264

19. Ludwig G (1991) Evaluation of conservative therapeutic approaches to Peyronie's disease (fibrotic induration of the penis). Urol Int 47:236–239
20. Devine CJ Jr, Horton CH (1974) Surgical treatment of Peyronie's disease with a dermal graft. J Urol 111:44–49
21. Ralph DJ, Brooks MD, Bottazzo GF, Pryor JP (1992) The treatment of Peyronie's disease with tamoxifen. Br J Urol 151:1522–1524
22. Levine LA, Merrick PF, Lee RC (1994) Intralesional verapamil injection for the treatment of Peyronie's disease. J Urol 151:1522–1524
23. Gelbard MK, James K, Riach P, Dorey F (1993) Collagenase versus placebo in the treatment of Peyronie's disease: a double-blind study. J Urol 149:56–58
24. Carson CC, Coughlin PW (1985) Radiation therapy for Peyronie's disease: is there a place? J Urol 134:684–686
25. Klevmark B, Andersen M, Schultz A, Talseth T (1994) Congenital and acquired curvature of the penis treated surgically by plication of the tunica albuginea. Br J Urol 74:501–506
26. Wild RM, Devine CJ, Horton CH (1979) Dermal graft repair of Peyronie's disease: survey of 50 patients. J Urol 121:47–50
27. Austoni E, Matovani F, Colombo F, Canclini L, Mastromarino G, Vecchio D, Fenice O (1994) Erectile complications after surgery for penile plastic induration. Arch Ital Urol Androl 66:19–22
28. Palomar JM, Halikiopoulos H, Thomas R (1980) Evaluation of the surgical management of Peyronie's disease. J Urol 123:680–682
29. Dalkin BL, Carter MF (1991) Venogenic impotence following dermal graft repair for Peyronie's disease. J Urol 146:849–851
30. Jones WJ Jr, Horton CE, Stecker JF Jr, Devine CJ Jr (1984) The treatment of psychogenic impotence after dermal graft repair for Peyronie's disease. J Urol 131:286–287
31. Malloy TR, Wein AJ, Carpiniello VL (1981) Advanced Peyronie's disease treated with the inflatable penile prosthesis. J Urol 125:327–328
32. Carson CC, Hodge GB, Anderson EE (1983) Penile prosthesis in Peyronie's disease. Br J Urol 417–421
33. Montorsi F, Guazzoni G, Bergamaschi F, Rigatti P (1993) Patient-partner satisfaction with semirigid penile prostheses for Peyronie's disease. J Urol 150:1819–1821
34. Kaufman JJ, Boxer B, Quinn MC (1981) Physical and psychological results of penile prostheses. J Urol 126:173

Priapism

V. GENTILE

Introduction

Priapism has been defined as a persistent erection, usually painful, and not necessarily associated with stimulation or sexual desire. Hinman (1960) defined priapism as hyperfunctioning of a mechanism which under normal basal conditions is physiologically reversible. This definition is inadequate in cases in which the patient has no penile sensibility, for example, following spinal injury or when an erection is provoked by the use of vasoactive substances, particularly in self-injection therapy.

The introduction of vasoactive agents in the diagnosis and treatment of erectile dysfunction has led to an increased incidence of iatrogenic priapism. Consequently, we consider it more appropriate to define priapism as a persistent erection of the penis for longer than 4–6 h (Broderick et al 1994).

Classification

As already pointed out, priapism may be spontaneous or iatrogenic. There are, in fact, two types of priapism, low-flow ischemic and high-flow nonischemic. The distinction between these being made on the basis of blood gas parameters and study of the penile blood flow.

The Erectile Mechanism

Observations on cadavers, monkeys, and dogs have shown that in the flaccid penis the smooth muscles of the corpus cavernosum and the helicine arteries are in a state of relative contraction. The neurotransmitters released during sexual stimulation induce relaxation of the smooth muscles of the trabecula and arteriolae, resulting in increased compliance of the sinusoidal system and consequently also the arterial flow. Expansion of the sinusoidal system in a limited space of the tunica albuginea compresses the venous plexus system which lies under the tunica and the emissary veins. The consequent transmission of the major part of the systolic pressure to the sinusoidal spaces transforms a flaccid penis into an erect one. Some neurotransmitters responsible for erection and for detumescence have recently (Saenz de Tejada 1988) been identified. Attention has focused on endothelial factors such as NO and VIP which induce relaxation of smooth muscle tissue, or endothelin which, on the other hand, leads to contraction of the smooth muscle, and the relationship of these factors with agents that block the α-adrenergic receptors, such as acetylcholine.

The Mechanism of Detumescence

Contraction of the smooth muscle of the vena cavernosa and arteriolae is probably provoked by an α-adrenergic discharge. The contraction of the sinusoidal smooth muscles leads to the opening of the venulae, thereby permitting a rapid discharge of blood from the corpora cavernosa. The arterial flow decreases, and gradually there is a return to normal of the arterial and venous flows causing the penis to return to a flaccid state. The neurotransmitter, endothelin, would appear, on account of the vasoconstrictive effect, to play an important role in this phase.

Etiopathogenesis

Some 35% of all cases of priapism are idiopathic, and 21% are associated with pharmacological therapy or with alcohol abuse. Other causes include perineal trauma (21%), falciform anemia (11%), and inflammatory diseases of the urogenital tract (8%). The relative distribution of the causes varies from report to report, geographical location, and age group. Other causes include leukemia, lipid embolisms, diabetic neuropathy, neoplastic infiltration of the penis, the use of antihypertensive drugs, and dialysis treatment. While there is much controversy regarding the causes of priapism, a widely accepted theory is that priapism results from injury to the mechanism that produces penile detumescence. This damage can be attributed to one of the following causes:

- Thromboembolytic factors: falciform anemia, drepanocytosis, leukemia, anticoagulant therapy, thromboembolic disorders, trauma, hematological disorders, neoplasms that involve the penis, and some local inflammatory process that impairs penile vein drainage, causing a persistent erection.
- Neurogenic factors (damage to the CNS, spinal cord, diabetic autonomic neuropathies, and a hyperactive sexual life): hyperstimulation of the erectile mechanism produces a constantly elevated blood flow in the penis resulting in high-flow priapism. Impairment of the mechanisms responsible for detumescence induces a closure of the venous mechanism causing a low-flow priapism.
- Drugs and other chemical substances taken orally (antidepressants, trazodone, chlorpromazine, thorazine, alcohol,and various others): more than likely these act upon the central and peripheral systems of tumescence or detumescence, causing a persistent erection.
- Vasoactive intracavernosal agents (papaverine, phenoxybenzamine, papaverine with phentolamine, prostaglandins, and others): when taken in large doses or inappropriately, some of these may lead to persistent erection. If the mechanisms of detumescence are not reactivated, priapism will ensue.

In some patients, priapism may resolve spontaneously even after it has been present for several days, and these patients recover the erectile potential. Others may become completely impotent after only 1–2 days of erectile tissue ischemia. Prognosis of these patients is determined by the grade of residual penile circulation and the state of the penis prior to priapism. In younger patients, restoration of erectile function is more likely. Electron microscope studies performed by Spycher and Hauri (1986) on erectile tissue after priapism have provided the first details of changes in the ultrastructure. In low-flow priapism the first reaction of the cavernosal tissue to modifications in the hemodynamic state is the formation of interstitial trabecular edema: 12 h after the onset of this condition, small defects in the cavernosal endothelium can be observed, while there is still no change in the smooth muscle cells of the cavernosum. After 12–14 h significant changes start with cytoplasmic transformations in the smooth muscle cells and progress to tissue necrosis. If the priapism persists for 24–48 h, there is widespread destruction of the sinusoidal endothelium, and the basal membrane becomes exposed. This leads to the adherence of thrombocytes with the formation of thrombi in the sinusoidal spaces, destruction of the endothelial membrane, and differentiation towards a fibroblastic condition.

The nerve fibers and their terminals accumulate neurotransmitters, and the blood capillaries display widespread tissue necrosis. In all the tissues examined, a combination of necrotic tissue and intact vascular structures is found. After a period of time, varying from several days to weeks, fibrosis begins to replace the cells initially present. It is not well known why or when the persistence of erection begins to cause irreversible damage. The damage to neuromuscular transmission and its functioning likely contributes to the irreversibility of the priapism.

Tissue specimens from two patients with high-flow priapism showed no structural changes despite the fact that when the biopsy was taken, the tumescence had been present for 14 days, in one case, and 5 months in the other (Havri et al. 1983).

Blood gases taken from inside the cavernosa start to show changes, due to the ischemia, 4–6 h after the onset of the priapism. The partial pressure of CO_2 increases from 39 to 55 mmHg, with a corresponding drop in pH to ≤ 7.31. If adequate therapy is not started for the priapism, these values do not return to normal, as generally occurs under physiological conditions.

Treatment

The aim of treatment in priapism is resolution of the painful symptoms, return to a normal flaccid state, and, above all, the preservation of normal erectile function. It is indispensable, when possible, to simultaneously treat the cause which triggered the condition. Various alternatives are available for treating priapism, and the choice depends upon how long the priapism has been present. We adhere to a well-defined outline based upon our own personal experience (Fig. 1) as well as that of others from all over the world. However, the therapy is often conditioned by the means available, considering the urgency involved in treating this condition (Ebbehoj 1975; Grayhack et al. 1964; Winter 1988).

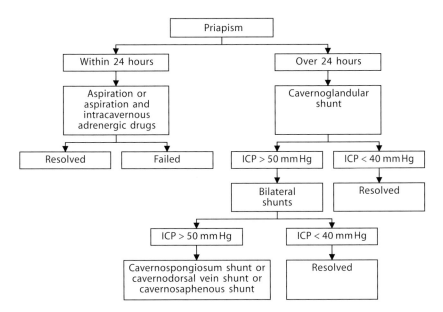

Fig. 1. Outline of treatment for priapism (ICP, intracavernous pressure)

It is fundamental, prior to deciding upon the type of treatment, to determine which of the two forms of priapism we are dealing with (Gentile et al. 1995). The time elapsed and mode of onset will emerge when collecting the patient's clinical history.

Blood gas aspirated from the corpora cavernosa should then be analyzed or, if available, sciniscan with 99-technetium, should be carried out. pH values < 7.25, $pO_2 < 30$ mmHg, and $pCO_2 > 60$ mmHg indicate the presence of ischemic priapism. Blood gas levels comparable to those of arterial blood are characteristic of high-flow priapism. In less frequent *nonischemic priapism* (arterial) following irrigation and aspiration from the corpora cavernosa, α-adrenergic drugs may be usefully employed, provided the patient has no evidence or history of cardiovascular disease. Should this procedure, however, be insufficient, then it will be necessary to proceed with one of the shunt or embolization techniques, the latter having been successfully adopted in nonischemic priapism. Selective arteriography is mandatory for embolization of the cavernous artery. It should not be forgotten that although only minimally invasive, embolization is not a harmless technique. Possible complications include penile gangrene, persistent impotence, and gluteal ischemia. In *ischemic priapism*, after aspiration and irrigation with a physiological solution, if less than 24 h have elapsed, it is possible to proceed with infusion of α-adrenergic drugs, various types of which have been used (phenylephrine, epinephrine, norepinephrine, ephredrine, dopamine). In contrast, if 24-36 h have elapsed, use of α-adrenergic drugs may induce an even more severe ischemia, whereas a shunt procedure would supply the oxygenated blood needed for functional restoration. The shunt procedures are the focal point of surgical treatment. The aim of the shunt is to create a new venous flow, thus increasing the gradient between the glans and the tip of the corpus cavernosum. Shunt procedures between corpora cavernosa and glans have been described by Chester Winter and Ebbejoh, the former using a biopsy needle, the latter a bistoury.

With the patient under general or local anesthesia, the glans is perforated with two large needles or with a biopsy needle, reaching into the corpora cavernosa. Clots and stagnant blood are aspirated until bright red blood appears. In order to keep the fistula open, tissue between the corpora cavernosa and the glans may be removed by means of a tru-cut which is rotated 360°. With Quackles'(Quackles 1964) technique, an anostomosis between the corpus cavernosum and corpus spongiosum of the urethra is created. This may be unilateral or bilateral depending upon the response obtained. Two matching flaps, 2 cm in length and l cm wide, between the corpus cavernosum and the corpus spongiosum are then anastomized. In the sapheno-cavernosa shunt described by Grayhack, corpus cavernosum blood is diverted directly into the systemic venous circulation through the saphenous vein.

The latter procedures are reserved for those cases in which the previously described shunts fail to resolve the priapism. The procedures described may lead to impotence in 50% of cases, more frequently with the cavernosum-spongiosum and sapheno-cavernosum shunts, even if this is often a direct consequence of the priapism itself.

Persistent Erection Induced by Vasoactive Drugs

The first step in reducing a persistent erection induced by vasoactive drugs is aspiration of blood from the corpora cavernosa if the erection has persisted for more than 4 h. Aspiration is performed with a butterfly with a 17- to 19-gauge needle. Detumescence generally follows after this simple procedure. It should be pointed out, however, that the problem may return within 1–2 h. If this procedure fails, we introduce 1 ml metaraminol 10% using the same butterfly: one vial in 10 cc saline solution, the administration of which can be repeated up to a maximum of 3 ml (1 ml every 15 min). A pediatric pressure cuff or pressure bandage may be used to compress the corpus cavernosum and thus maintain venous drainage. This procedure can be performed even when priapism, induced by vasoactive drugs, has been present for hours; however, there is less chance of success. Patients with erectile dysfunction of neurogenic origin require constant monitoring since they tend to develop repeated episodes of tumescence even after three or four aspirations.

The persistence of erectile dysfunction beyond 3 months should be investigated by means of cavernospongiography, which can provide useful information concerning the trabecular system, fibrosis, and the condition of the shunt (Bondil 1990; Lue et al. 1986).

Discussion

One of the major controversies regarding the treatment of priapism is when to operate. Priapism is usually considered a surgical emergency. Spycher and Hauri, on the basis of electron microscope studies, recommend that patients with ischemic priapism be operated on during the first 24 h, before changes occur in the smooth muscle (Spycher and Hauri 1986; Hauri et al. 1983).

Younger patients probably have a higher recovery rate due to the better condition of their vascular system and the cavernosum tissue; however, this should not be a reason to delay treatment in these patients.

In patients with a suspected relapse of priapism during the postoperative period, blood-gas analysis may help in making a differential diagnosis between tumescence due to tissue edema (normal blood gas levels) and a relapse (ischemic blood gas levels). Monitoring the intracavernosum pressure we can: (a) confirm the diagnosis, (b) evaluate the efficiency of the intracavernosum α-adrenergic agents or the condition of the shunt, and (c) determine the end-point of the procedure. We consider Winter's procedure, preferable to others, as it is more practical and efficacious; only when this does not work should Quackles' procedure (cavernospongiosum shunt) be considered.

However, in patients with severe ischemia and priapism that lasts for more than 24 h, a shunt must be created that provides immediate revascularization of the tissues. In this situation, an α-adrenergic agent could worsen the situation.

For practical purposes, priapism induced by intracavernosum injections of vasoactive drugs can be divided into two different categories: (a) priapism which has been present for less than 6 h responds well to aspiration treatment alone or aspiration treatment plus the use of injections of α-adrenergic drugs, and (b) priapism resulting from an injection lasting for more than 12 h must be treated in the same manner as for the other types of priapism.

References

1. Bondil P (1990) Aspects physiopathologiques du priapisme. J Urol 96(2):115–118
2. Broderick GA, Gordon D, Hypolite J, Levin RM (1994) Anoxia and corporal smooth muscle dysfunction: a model for ischemic priapism. J Urol 151:259–262
3. Ebbehoj J (1975) A new operation for priapism. Scand J Plast Reconstr Surg 8:241–242
4. Gentile V, Prigiotti G, La Pera G, Di Palma P (1995) La terapia chirurgica del priapism. G Ital Androl 2:87–91
5. Grayhack J, McCullough W, O'Connor V Jr et al. (1964) Venous bypass to control priapism. Invest Urol 1:509–513
6. Hauri D, Spycher M, Bruhlmann V (1983) Erection and priapism: a new pathophysiological concept. Urol Int 38:138–145
7. Hinman F Jr (1960) Priapism: reasons for failure of therapy. J Urol 83:420–428
8. Lue T, Hellstrom WJG, McAnic JW, Tanagho EA (1986) Priapism: a refined approach to diagnosis and treatment. J Urol 136:104–107
9. Quackles R (1964) Cure of a patient suffering from priapism by cavernoso-sponsgiosal anastomosis. Acta Urol Belg 32:5
10. Saenz de Tejada I, Goldstein I, Krane RJ (1988) Local control of penile erection. Nerves, smooth muscle and endothelium. Urol Clin N Am 15:9
11. Spycher MA, Hauri D (1986) The ultrastructure of the erectile tissue in priapism. J Urol 135:142–147
12. Winter CC (1978) Priapism cured by creation of fistulas between glans penis and corpora cavernosa. J Urol 119:227–228
13. Winter CC (1988) Experience with 105 patients with priapism: up–date review of all aspects. J Urol 140:980–983

Part II

Varicocele

Varicocele: "A Never Ending Story"

F. Menchini Fabris

Since Pare's definition of varicocele in the year 1500 as "a mass of melancholy blood," the problem of a correlation between venous scrotal ectasiae and fertility impairment has continued the subject of controversy. Still today the surgical correction of varicose veins is considered by many andrologists indispensable for functional reestablishment of spermatogenesis, while this is denied by others. There are indeed many different approaches to the problem of infertility in men, and there are too many aspects of the problem to allow a standardization of criteria and the establishment of indications for the surgical treatment of varicocele. The legitimate question of the patient is always the same: "Will the procedure be useful or not?"

Regardless of the surgical technique, however, the factors with predictive power for evaluating the feasibility of surgery are:

- The age of the patient is a fundamental factor in the evaluation of the varicocele because it is correlated to the damage suffered by the testis during the exposure to varicocele.
- The testicular volume is directly proportional to a spermatogenesis. Two-thirds of the testicular volume consists of the tubular part.
- The monolaterality or bilaterality of varicocele is a factor of great prognostic significance. A bilateral varicocele can even cause an azoospermia, which can regress after the surgical correction of spermatic veins.
- The grade of varicocele can be evaluated using different methods. It is also a very important prognostic factor.
- The endocrine evaluation and particularly the level of follicle-stimulating hormone can provide significant information about spermatogenesis.

- The spermatogenesis is obviously very important but can present great changes in few years. The correlation must always be assessed to the volume of the testis and to the patient's age.
- Sperm morphology is central in evaluating the ejaculate of a patient with varicocele. In these patients the proportion of normal sperms does not exceed 40%. In addition, they show head anomalies. The reduction of these head anomalies over a period of 3–6 months after surgical correction is very significant to the success of the treatment (Menchini Fabris et al. 1985).

However, the following steps are essential: (a) an accurate diagnosis, obtained by an echo color Doppler, (b) a detailed sperm evaluation with a particular attention to the morphology of spermatozoa, (c) some pharmacological therapy (after 3–6 months of the surgical correction) supporting the functional reestablishment of spermatogenesis, and (d) a common flow-sheet for the various specialists who attend infertile patients with varicocele. Under these conditions, the never-ending story of varicocele will find a conclusion.

Reference

Menchini Fabris GF, Canale D, Basile Fasolo C, Di Coscio M, Izzo PL, Giannotti P, Marino P, Servadio L, Baldassarri S, Fratta M (1985) Varicocele and male subfertility: prognostical criteria in the surgical treatment. Andrologia 17:16–21

Varicocele: Diagnosis

A. Ledda, G. Belcaro, G. Laurora, and A. Bottari

Introduction

The varicocele is the most widespread andrological pathology and also the most frequent cause of infertility in men. On average it affects about 15% of the male population; however, this increases to 39% among the patients who seek help in andrological centers for infertility problems [1]. Dilatation of the scrotal vein due to valvular incompetence in the pampiniform plexus (and/or in the spermatic veins) reduces the venous return in the scrotum, causing a stagnation of blood and thus increasing the testicular temperature. Testicular hyperthermia in turn reduces the number of spermatozoa, decreases their motility, and alters their morphology, which manifests itself as an increased number of spermatozoa at an immature stage. The sequence of pathological events determined by the scrotal venous return initially produces a venous hypertension which is followed by edema. These factors cause a predisposition to scrotal hyperthermia [2]. The damage resulting from scrotal hyperthermia includes testicular hypotrophy and oligospermia, which tend to deteriorate while the hyperthermia persists. It is therefore important to ascertain all the alterations present in patients with varicoceles, obviously starting with an analysis of the seminal fluid, by means of a sperm count, followed by a complete echographic work-up.

As described in detail elsewhere in this volume, the "gold standard" for diagnosis of varicocele is a retrograde phlebogram of the spermatic vein. This, however, should not be a prime consideration in the initial work-up. Other, less invasive procedures should first be considered. This examination and the Valsalva-Ivanissevich maneuver cannot confirm the presence of a subclinical varicocele, it is therefore always a good practice to resort to an ultrasound examination, which can visualize the veins and measure venous return. When the patient is in an orthostatic position, the scrotal veins have a maximum diameter of about 4 mm. In normal patients the scrotal veins, as is common for all peripheral veins, show either a modest venous return, or this is completely absent following an increase in pressure resulting from a Valsalva maneuver, or when pressure is applied manually. In patients with a varicocele the transverse diameter of the vein can be as wide as 9–10 mm.

The use of ultrasonography (echography or Doppler) has been shown to be valuable for evaluating varicoceles and all other pathological scrotal conditions including lesions resulting from trauma, ischemia, neoplasms, and inflammation. The recent introduction of echo color Doppler has greatly decreased the time necessary to evaluate the vascular, morphological, and volumetric status of the testicles. With the advent of color Doppler both the direction and velocity of scrotal blood flow can easily be determined and measured (Figs. 1a-d) [4,5,7,8]. In just a few minutes this noninvasive procedure provides all the information that until a few years ago required more invasive examinations (e.g., phlebography or a scintigraphy). The testicular evaluation with this technique is extremely detailed. Placing these images over those obtained with the classical gray scale echography permits immediate interpretation of the pathological situation as well as the measurement of blood flow. This information should be correlated with the clinical findings and then completed with a thermographic evaluation. These results serve as a reference for comparison to those obtained postoperatively or after scleroembolization of the spermatic veins. A diagnostic evaluation using echo color Doppler is commonly known as an angiodynography because it visualizes as well as measures vascular flow [3].

Scrotal Angiodynographic Technique

In 1988 a study was begun using angiodynography to diagnose patients suffering from varicoceles. The patients were divided into two groups: those in whom the varicocele was clinically evident and those patients in whom the varicocele (subclinical) could be diagnosed only by relying upon diagnostic examinations and was associated with oligospermia

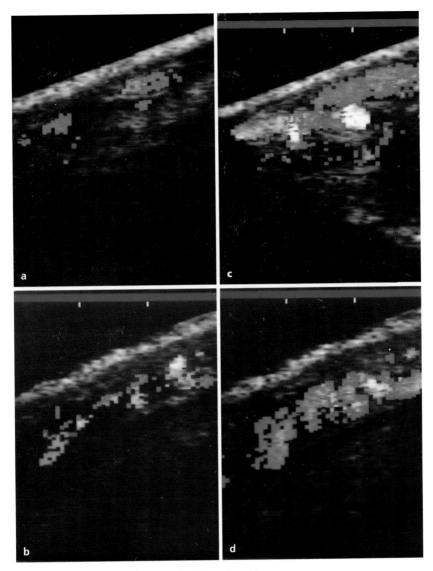

Fig. 1 a-d. Scrotal echo color Doppler (four phases)

and/or asymmetry of the testicles. The evaluation was by echo Doppler ATL Mark 8 with an 10-MHz probe and with an echo color Doppler Quantum (Philips) with a 7.5-MHz probe and a Bruel and Kjaer 3535 with a 7.5-MHz probe at high resolution.

The examination begins with visualization of the spermatic vein while the patient is in a supine position. A small spontaneous reflux that is associated with respiration is sometimes observed. The patient is then asked to perform a Valsalva maneuver, which accentuates the reflux if present. Examining the veins during the period of maximum reflux permits a quantitative measurement to be obtained. The flow is proportional to the velocity multiplied by the area of a transverse section of the vein. The average reflux can also be measured; this is proportional to the area under the curve. The Valsalva maneuver is repeated at least three times to obtain a reliable reading. The patient is normally evaluated in a supine position; however, if the venous return cannot be visualized, the patient is asked to assume an erect position. The supine rather than erect position is preferred for the examination because there is less abdominal muscular tension with the patient in a supine position, and this permits scanning under more natural conditions and produces fewer artifacts.

The dimensions of the largest spermatic veins during the Valsalva maneuver were measured using the technique described by Orda et al. [6]. The peak velocity of venous flow and the average venous return during the first 3 s of the Valsalva maneuver were also measured. The methodology of the results obtained with the color Doppler were compared (in specifically selected patients) with those obtained by means of a retrograde phlebogram of the spermatic veins. We excluded from this study both those patients who were not able to perform the Valsalva maneuver correctly and those who had undergone previous surgery on the spermatic veins or other pathological conditions involving the spermatic cord or scrotum. Table 1 shows the characteristics of the patients considered in this study; there was no significant age difference between the two groups nor between them and the control group. Table 2 shows the maximum diameter of the spermatic cord vein (MVD), the peak velocity (PFV) recorded with the echo color Doppler and the average venous return obtained during the maneuver of Valsalva.

A significant difference was found between the MVD of patients with subclinical or clinical varicoceles and that of the control group during the Valsalva maneuver. Patients with subclinical varicocele had a PFV of 18 cm/s, which was significantly lower than the reflux found in patients with a clinically detectable varicocele. Separating the patients with a clinically visible varicocele from those with a subclinical case, we formed three subgroups: (a) reflux of under 3 s during the Valsalva maneuver, (b) reflux of 3–5 s during the Valsalva maneuver, and (c) reflux of over

Table 1. Details of normal subjects and of patients with clinical and subclinical varicoceles

Patients	Number	Mean	SD	Range
Subclinical	107	26	7	12 – 24
Clinical	228	27	6	13 – 40
Normal	22	26	5	14 – 30

Table 2. Maximum venous diameters, peak flow velocities, and mean reflux during Valsalva maneuver

Varicocele	Maximum venous diameter during Valsalva maneuver (cm)	Reflux Peak flow velocity	Reflux Mean reflux in 3 s
Subclinical	0.34	18	0.8
Clinical	0.66	24	4.1
Normals	0.1 – 0.2	< 10	–

Table 3. Classification of patients in three groups according to the duration of reflux and comparing the peak flow velocities in the spermatic veins during a Valsalva maneuver

Varicocele	< 3 s	> 3s < 5 s	> 5s
Subclinical mean (cm/S)	14	18.5	20
SD	6	7	7
Clinical mean (cm/S)	19.2	24.3	28
SD	7	9	8

Table 4. Percent distribution of patients according to the duration of venous testicular reflux (evaluated by echo color Doppler)

Varicocele	< 3 s (%)	> 3s < 5 s (%)	> 5s (%)
Subclinical	5	80	15
Clinical	1	69	30

5 s. The relative PFV can be observed in the three subgroups (Table 3). The PFV was a significantly higher in patients with clinical varicoceles, accompanied by an increase in the PFV in the three subgroups, in the clinical as well as the subclinical form. Table 4 illustrates the percentage of cases with varicoceles in relation to the subgroup classification. In the group with subclinical varicoceles only 5% had a reflux shorter than 3 s,

80% had a reflux time between 3 and 5 s, and the remaining 15% showed a reflux longer than 5 s. In the clinical cases only 1% had a reflux time under 3 s, in 69% of patients the reflux time was between 3 and 5 s; and in the remaining 30% it was above 5 s.

Discussion

A noninvasive diagnostic evaluation of a varicocele can be obtained by many techniques. However, none of these techniques are perfect. Even echography has been proposed for studying varicoceles [6]. This technique is limited to defining the dimensions of the individual veins of the spermatic cord, and obviously it is an excellent screening method for varicoceles. However, it does not provide a quantitative evaluation, and often it is very difficult to use if the patient has undergone surgery or sclerotherapy. An echo color Doppler examination is easy to perform and interpret and provides a very precise quantitative evaluation of the venous return, determining the caliber of the vein, PFV, and average venous return during the Valsalva maneuver. However, it is important to point out that a quantitative evaluation of the reflux is not always possible, and that if it is, it requires a considerable amount of time, in contrast to the qualitative demonstration of reflux which is a very simple and effective examination that can be performed in a matter of minutes. In addition to the ease with which this examination can be performed, another important advantage is the ability to clearly show the patient his problem.

In conclusion, the scrotal echo color Doppler is particularly useful for diagnosing the presence of a varicocele, not only for studying the individual patient but also for comparing, in a very precise manner, the results of various therapeutic techniques such as surgery, microsurgery, and all the other methods that employ sclerotherapeutic agents.

Conclusion

Diagnostic methods using ultrasonography are now refined and reliable and can present a precise picture of any hemodynamic alterations. This information must always be considered together with the clinical picture of the patient and from the other parameters of testicular function. The combination of all this information directs the physician towards a decision as to the most appropriate therapy in particularly difficult cases, and this is often the problem when adolescents are involved. It is much easier to select the type of treatment when confronted with a case of infertility that does not involve any other identifiable causes. The sensitivity and sensibility of these new techniques can eliminate many problems, especially in the case of a subclinical varicocele.

The criteria for surgery have been widely discussed from an ethical standpoint because in many cases it might seem to be forced upon the patient. In the beginning Dubin and Amelar [1] and subsequently McClure [9] have shown that the presence of a subclinical varicocele provokes the same testicular damage as the clinical form. In addition, a diagnosis based upon ultrasonography permits an early diagnosis in adolescents. Various experts in the field have emphasized the importance of early diagnosis to protect their fertility later. Various studies have shown that treatment of varicoceles in adolescents can increase their potential fertility. Echography, Doppler, and color Doppler are indispensable diagnostic tools that give the physician an excellent overall clinical picture of the patient by enabling him to determine testicular volume and evaluate the scrotal hemodynamic situation. In addition, it is possible to obtain an adequate follow-up, which is especially important in younger patients who are more prone to testicular hypotrophy.

References

1. Dubin L, Amelar RD (1971) Etiology factors in 1294 consecutive cases of male infertility. Fert Steril 22:469–474
2. Zorgniotti AW, MacLeod J (1973) Studies in temperature, human semen quality and varicocele. Fertil Steril 24:854–863
3. Ledda A, Belcaro G (1991) Assessment of varicocele with angiodynography (color-coded triplex). Vasc Surg 25(7):559–564
4. Middleton WD, Thorne DA, Melson GL (1989) Color Doppler ultrasound of normal testis. AJR Am J Roentgenol 152:293–297
5. Lerner RM, Mevorach RA, Hulbert WC et al (1990) Color Doppler ultrasound in the evaluation of acute scrotal disease. Radiology 176:355–358
6. Orda R, Sayfan J, Manor H et al (1987) Diagnosis of varicocele a post-operative evaluation using inguinal ultrasonography. Ann Surg 206:99–101
7. Greenberg SH, Lipshultz LI, Morganroth J, Wein AJ (1977) The use of the Doppler stethoscope in the evaluation of varicoceles. J Urol 117:296–298
8. Hirsch AV, Cameron KM, Tyler JP, Simpson J, Pryor JP (1980) The Doppler assessment of varicoceles and internal spermatic vein reflux in infertile men. Br J Urol 52:50–56
9. McClure RD, Khoo D, Jarvi K, Hricak H (1991) Subclinical varicocele: the effectiveness of varicocelectomy. J Urol 145:789–791

Percutaneous Sclerotherapy of Internal Spermic Veins

C. Trombetta, M. Deriu, E. Salisci, and E. Belgrano

Introduction

The importance of varicocele as a correctable cause of male infertility has been confirmed by several studies. Many authors have reported the recovery of spermatogenesis in azoospermic patients by varicocele ligation, and an increasing number of studies have reported the association of varicocele with testicular atrophy and infertility. Varicocele is the commonest cause of male infertility although only one of five men with varicocele is infertile. Although it is still unclear what mechanisms are involved in the dysfunction resulting from varicocele, it has been demonstrated that varicocele correction leads to an improvement in the quality of semen in most cases.

The standard surgical procedure for varicocele correction is the ligature of internal spermatic veins; however, in about 10%–25% of the cases the varicocele persists after this surgical intervention. A routine preoperative phlebographic study of the varicocele by left spermatic vein selective catherization has been advocated by several authors. This provides information in advance about the characteristics of the veins to be ligated and helps to establish the etiology of the varicocele and its proper management. Therefore venography has become a routine diagnostic tool for varicocele, followed by its outgrowth, transcatheter sclerotherapy of varicocele. We review here our experience in a venographic study and transcatheter sclerotherapy based on 560 cases of infertile patients with varicocele (Fig. 1).

Fig. 1. Left renography: presence of a large spermatic vein

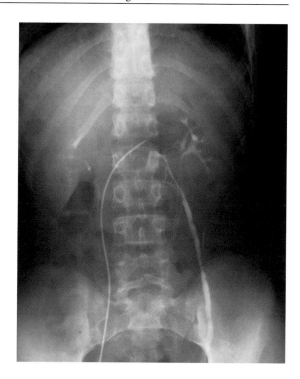

Material and Methods

A total of 560 infertile patients with varicocele have received percutaneous scleroembolization since 1986 in our institute [1]. All patients underwent diagnostic preoperative evaluation by repeated semen analyses, Doppler flowmetry, scrotal ultrasound, and venography. Data from preoperative semen analyses are summarized in Table 1. Venography is performed through the transfemoral approach under local anesthesia on an outpatient basis (Fig. 2). A 6-F C₃ femoral-visceral catheter is commonly used to catheterize the renal vein selectively. Renal phlebography is carried out by the injection of 20 ml of contrast medium under Valsalva maneuver with the patient in standing position. The catheter is then changed for another endhole one for selective catheterization of the left spermatic vein. Once the vein has been cannulated, a spermatic

Table 1. Preoperative seminal findings (n=560)

	Percentage
Number	
$<5 \times 10^6$	17,5
$5 - 10 \times 10^6$	20.6
$10 - 20 \times 10^6$	19.0
$20 - 30 \times 10^6$	14.3
$30 - 40 \times 10^6$	9.5
$40 - 50 \times 10^6$	7.9
$>50 \times 10^6$	11.1
Motility (2h)	
<10%	14.8
10% – 20%	32.5
20% – 30%	11.5
30% – 40%	13.1
40% – 50%	11.5
50% – 60%	4.9
>60%	11.7
Morphology[a]	
<10%	1.7
10% – 20%	10.3
20% – 30%	15.5
30% – 40%	21.1
40% – 50%	12.3
50% – 60%	12.1
60% – 70%	10.3
>70%	13.7

[a] percentage of normal sperms.

phlebography is obtained by injecting 5 ml 50% diluted contrast medium. To avoid total radiation exposure the testicles should be shielded by a capsule and the number of roentgenograms restricted to a minimum of 1 or 2.

Scrotal ultrasound was performed in 310 patients to evaluate the echogenicity of the testes, their volume, and funicular vein enlargement during Valsalva maneuver. Relative hypotrophy of the testis in the presence of varicocele was encountered in almost all cases. In 2 patients operated on for cryptorchism there was a contralateral smaller testicle.

Fig. 2. A distal scleroembolization has been
achieved: dye is stopping
in the spermatic vein

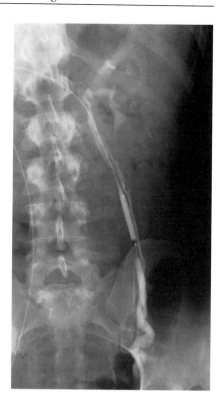

Scleroembolization Technique

Scleroembolization is performed when the etiologic factor of varicocele
arises in the presence of stasis into the left renal vein with consequent
renospermatic reflux and reversal of the direction of blood flow within
the spermatic vein. The venous hypertension is a result of the left renal
vein compression by the angle formed posteriorly by the abdominal
aorta and anteriorly by the take off of the superior mesenteric artery,
forming the so-called "high nut-cracker". After selective catheterization
of the spermatic vein, a guide wire is introduced deeply into the vein, and
the first catheter is replaced by a smaller one previously curved for this
purpose. This catheter permits very distal catheterization. The optimal
level for scleroembolization is at the ilium because here the ureter is
further from the spermatic vessels. Scleroembolization is performed by
injecting 4–8 ml Trombovar (3%) and 50% glucose solution in water into

the spermatic vein. Before injecting the substances we usually damage the intima by means of the guide wire. We routinely repeat the scleroembolization at two levels. In some cases when very dilated veins are present, a balloon catheter is used. When ethanol is used as sclerotizing agent, an external clamping of the funicular structures prevents testicular damage. Scleroembolization is continued until complete occlusion of the vein has been achieved, with stagnation of the contrast medium. The whole procedure lasts 30–45 min; the average cost of the scleroembolization is US-$ 900 (1996).

Results

Venographic evaluation was possible in 97.8% of all cases. In 15 patients who were not included in this study, a selective catheterization of internal spermatic vein was not possible. In 2% of the cases a deep catheterization was not possible, and in 2% renospermatic reflux was not evident. Left iliac phlebography revealed in these patients an iliac stasis (the patients were operated on and are not included in these data; Figs. 3-5). Postoperative Doppler flowmetry showed the persistence of the venous reflux in 17.1% of the patients who underwent scleroembolization and had already been operated on. All these patients showed the persistence of a clear renospermatic reflux at venography. Venographic findings (375 patients/560 veins as follows:

- Number of veins: one, 118; two, 67; three or more, 190
- Presence of two renal veins: 19 (5.4%)
- Circumaortic ring: 34 (9.7%)
- Presence of anastomosis with vena porta: 8 (2.2%)
- Presence of two complete and separate veins: 18 (5.1%)

Three months after scleroembolization semen analyses were repeated. An increase in the number of sperms was found in 87.7% of the cases (in 41% of these the number was doubled). We evaluated the percentage of motile sperms at 2 h, and in 70% of the cases an increase was evident. The percentage of morphologically normal sperms increased in 81% of

Fig. 3. Presence of a rare anastomosis with the mesenteric vein

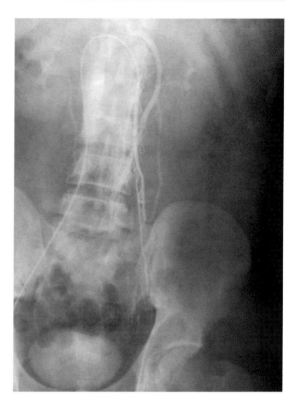

the cases. Pregnancy of the partner followed scleroembolization in 33.7% (follow-up: 6 months–8 years).

We are evaluating testicular sizes by means of ultrasound. We do not yet have sufficient data to make definitive conclusions, but a certain increase in testicular size in younger patients is already evident.

Complications

There have been no major complications directly related to venography or scleroembnolization. One case of hematuria and two cases of phlebitis of the spermatic plexus have been encountered. In the majority of cases the only side effect is moderate inguinal or lumbar pain for 3–4 h. The list of side effects and complications encountered in 375 patients is as follows:

Fig. 4. After having sclerotized the medial vein, two collateral veins sustain renospermatic reflux

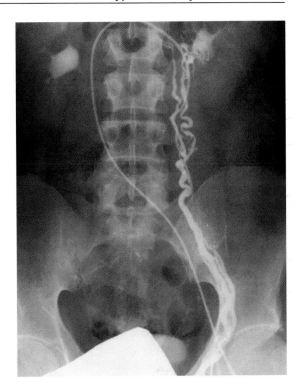

- Hematuria: 1
- Phlebitis of the spermatic plexus: 2
- Hematoma in the site of puncture: 15
- Fever (38 °C): 22
- Slight contrast medium reaction: 12
- Lumbar pain (24 h): 5

Discussion

An increasing number of men are asking the urologist for correction of varicocele to treat or prevent infertility. Since most are young and healthy, and the procedure is elective, it would be better to develop a technique that entails minimal risks and provides an inexpensive solution to the problem. The risks of percutaneous scleroembolization are actually minimal as the procedure can be performed entirely under local anesthesia at the site of venipuncture. We have observed no major complications in our series, and no major complication has been reported in the literature.

The effectiveness of scleroembolization must be related to the correct indications and to the persistence of the venous occlusion. The diagnosis of reflux in these patients is documented by renal venography in standing position. In the angiographic visualization of the renospermatic reflux, it must be taken into consideration that simple occlusion of the internal spermatic vein, according to the technique of Ivanissevich, does not provide complete resolution of varicocele in all cases. This can be explained by the different pathogenetic mechanisms which lead finally to hypertension in the spermatic plexus and varicose dilation of the spermatic veins.

Venography is the only method that can show all the aspects of the hemodynamic situation of varicocele. Doppler flowmetry gives evidence only of renospermatic reflux during the Valsalva maneuver and cannot demonstrate iliac hypertension (which is responsible for about 2%–5% of varicocele) or the number and the size of the veins.

In the case of renospermatic reflux, by far the most common cause of varicocele, venous hypertension comes from the renal vein, and causes a reflux into the internal spermatic vein. Occlusion of the internal spermatic vein is mandatory, and in many cases this is enough to solve the problem because venous drainage through the external spermatic veins into the iliac vein is efficient. Occlusion of the internal spermatic vein can be carried out out by surgical ligation or by percutaneous therapy. Our results show that scleroembolization is more efficient than high surgical ligation in removing renospermatic reflux.

Scleroembolization entails no additional cost with respect to diagnostic venography and can be carried whenever selective and distal catheterization of the internal spermatic vein has been achieved [3-6]. In addition, the cost of scleroembolization in terms of eventual complications is extremely low so that the procedure can be planned on an outpatient basis. On the other hand, we believe that embolization of the internal spermatic vein, carried out with a Gianturco-Anderson metal coil as suggested by Thelen (1979) is too dangerous for use in eliminating a cause of infertility; the risk of pulmonary embolism due to coil mobilization is very high.

On the basis of our experimental and clinical experience we do not consider cyanoacrylates as suitable for venous embolization because (a) they always require a balloon catheter, (b) the balloon can be entrapped by the polymerizing embolus, and (c) a minimal mistake can provoke a lethal pulmonary embolism.

In conclusion, we feel that scleroembolization offers a better cost-benefit ratio than surgery and should be the first-choice treatment of varicocele when renospermatic reflux is present. In cases of technically impossible selective catheterization of spermatic vein (Fig. 5) we prefer to plan microsurgical intervention of spermaticoepigastric anastomosis [2]. When scleroembolization proves unsuccessful, an antegrade percutaneous therapy can be performed with the technique proposed by Tauber.

Fig. 5. Anomalous venous circulation: kidney capsular venous circulation is widely connected with left spermatic vein, and distal catheterization is technically impossible

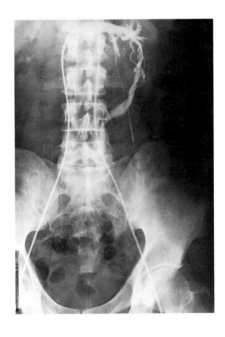

References

1. Belgrano E, Puppo P, Quattrini S, Trombetta C, Giuliani L (1984a) The role of venography and sclerotherapy in the management of varicocele. Eur Urol 10:124–129

2. Belgrano E, Puppo P, Gaboardi F, Trombetta C (1984b) A new microsurgical technique for varicocele correction. J Androl 5:148–154

3. Bigat JM, Chatel A (1980) The value of retrograde spermatic phlebography in varicocele. Eur Urol 6:301–306

4. Coolsaet BLRA (1980) The varicocele syndrome: venography determining the optimal level for surgical management. J Urol 124:833–839

5. Riedl P (1979) Selektive Phlebographie und Katheterthrombosierung der Vena testicularis bei primärer Varicocele. Wien Med Wochenschr 91 [Suppl]:89

6. Thelen M, Weissbach L, Franken T (1979) Die Behandlung der idiopatischen Varikozele durch transfemorale Spiralokklusion der Vena testicularis sinistra. Fortschr Geb Röntgstr Nuklearmed Erganzungsbd 131:24–29

Videolaparoscopic Spermatic Veins Ligation in Cases of Bilateral Varicocele

C. Trombetta, M. Deriu, and E. Salisci

Introduction

The laparoscopic treatment of varicocele has been proposed by several authors [1–3]. This new technique has increased the already considerable divergence of opinion about the ideal method of varicocele correction. Laparoscopic spermatic vein ligation is based on the high ligation method, whose percentage of recurrences is due to the presence of venous collaterals [4, 5].

Since 1979 we have emphasized the role of phlebography especially in infertile patients [6] because knowledge of the collateral circulation is important for obtaining a successful radiological treatment. Today, we treat left varicocele successfully by sclerotherapy today in more than 98% of cases. The use of scrotal ultrasound in infertile men in recent years has increased the detection of bilateral varicoceles [7]. In bilateral cases we have adopted both percutaneous treatment (with a success rate of 70%) and microsurgery [8]. In the last 5 years for cases of bilateral varicocele we have preferred laparoscopy as treatment, which offers substantial advantages over the classical surgical technique. In cases of bilateral varicocele a laparoscopic operation requires no second incision and minimally increases the operative time. Postoperative discomfort is decreased significantly compared to that in traditional surgery, allowing the patient to return to normal activity much sooner. We describe below our procedures for laparoscopic treatment of bilateral varicocele in a group of 22 patients who were followed for 6 months after the procedure.

Material and Methods

Patient Selection

Twenty-two men aged 22–38 years (mean 32 years) underwent bilateral laparoscopic spermatic vein ligation. The diagnosis of varicocele was based on physical examination and Doppler flowmetry of funicular veins and arteries; testicular volume was measured by scrotal ultrasound. Indications for an operation included infertility in 19 patients and the presence of repeated semen analyses showing a stress sperm pattern in three (one of whom reported left scrotal pain). One patient had already been operated on at another hospital at the inguinal level for a left varicocele. At the time of our observation he had a grade II right varicocele and a grade III left recurrent varicocele. No patient reported a history of extensive bowel adhesions with peritonitis or concomitant intestinal obstruction. One of them had undergone appendectomy, with no postoperative complication. We do not consider obesity to be a contraindication to laparoscopic varix ligation, although special care is to be taken in obese patients during insertion of the insufflating needle and establishment of the pneumoperitoneum. A preoperative abdominal ultrasound is always performed to rule out the presence of any unsuspected pathology, such as aortic aneurysms, urachal cysts, and solid masses.

Patient Preparation

All laparoscopic procedures are performed with the patient under general anesthesia. The patient is placed in the Trendelenburg position to displace the bowels toward the head. During the intervention it may be convenient to rotate the patient to the right or left side to facilitate cord identification. A wide area of the skin is prepared in the standard fashion (including shaving and application of a topical antibacterial agent) extending from the subcostal margin to the middle thigh, lateral to the posterior axillary lines, and including the scrotum. The testicles may be tugged during the procedure to aid in identifying the testicular vessels. A Foley catheter is always inserted to empty the bladder. The nasogastric tube is aspirated before the Veress needle is passed into the peritoneal cavity.

An initial 1-cm incision is made subumbilically in the midline and carried down to the fascia. The abdominal wall is retracted away from the intraperitoneal contents. The Veress needle is inserted into the peritoneum through an umbilical incision and directed toward the pelvis. One must feel that the needle has passed two points of palpable resistance (the fascia and the peritoneum). Sterile saline (10 ml) is dripped into the needle to ensure proper placement. The return of saline during aspiration suggests preperitoneal placement of the Veress needle.

Pneumoperitoneum

The needle is then connected to a positive flow of carbon dioxide which is instilled at a rate of 1 l/min. The intraperitoneal pressure is monitored in real time by a pressure transducer and should be low (less than 5 mmHg) at the start of insufflation. The peritoneal cavity in men is distended with approximately 4.5–6 l gas; during intervention to maintain a pressure of 10–14 mmHg is maintained. The monitor of the pump must be observed throughout the procedure to control the intra-abdominal pressure and the total volume of the carbon dioxide that has been used.

Insertion of the Trocars

Once adequate pneumoperitoneum has been obtained, the Veress needle is removed, and the 10-mm laparoscopic trocar is introduced through the same site. Once the trocar and sheath have entered the peritoneal cavity an audible escape of CO_2 gas is heard through the trocar channel. A full-beam video camera is attached to the ocular piece of the laparoscope which is passed through the sheath. The abdominal contents are examined to confirm placement within the peritoneal cavity. The CO_2 insufflation is resumed through the sheath channel to maintain the pneumoperitoneum with an intraperitoneal pressure of 10–14 mmHg. If only one monitor is available, it can be positioned at the foot of the operating table. We have extensive experience with the simultaneous use of two monitors placed in front of the two operators.

In addition to the laparoscope insertion site, three additional working ports are required to provide access for operating instruments in cases of bilateral varicocele. An 11-mm access port is positioned through the linea alba midway between the umbilicus and pubic symphysis. Then we use two 5.5-mm working ports in the inferolateral position inserted medially with respect to the ipsilateral anterior iliac spine (Fig. 1). Before trocar insertion the laparoscope is positioned near each insertion site to illuminate the abdominal wall and control the intraperitoneal contents beneath the insertion site.

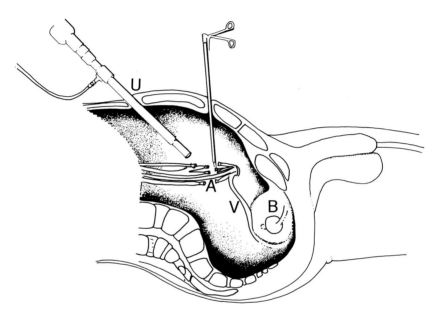

Fig. 1. Laparoscopy of varicocele: the videocamera is inserted through umbilical trocar (*U*). Veins (*V*) are twice clipped and divided. Division of the veins facilitates exposure and preservation of the artery (*A*). *B*, bladder

Dissection

After any necessary lysis of adhesions the anatomy is usually clear, with the testicular vessels advancing towards the internal ring to be joined by the vas deferens and its associated vessels. With a careful dissecting technique the posterior peritoneum overlying the testicular vessels is incised with the laparoscopic scissors. The operator stands on the contralateral side of the operating table and manipulates the midline and ipsilateral instrument (scissors with the right hand and curved hemostats with the left hand). The assistant, who can operate the contralateral varicocele, must deal with a mirror-image frame of reference; in any case he can help the operator by using straight hemostats or irrigation-suction devices.

A Hagood incision [2] is performed 0.5–1 cm anterior to the spermatic vessels and 1–2 cm from the vas. Donovan and Winfield [3] recommend a 5-cm peritoneal incision parallel and lateral to the spermatic vessels; the medial peritoneal edge of the incision is grasped, and a second peritoneal incision is made at a right angle to the first extending medially over the spermatic vessels to produce a T incision and expose the lateral and medial borders of the spermatic vascular pocket. We have used both techniques but now prefer only one 5- to 6-cm peritoneal incision parallel and lateral to the spermatic vessels as this is sufficient to elevate and to compartmentalize the cord by a curved dissector. The artery is usually found posteriorly and medially. Dissection can cause spasm in the artery; however, by irrigating the area with a few drops of papaverine or lidocaine the pulse generally returns and is visible or detectable by intraoperative Doppler ultrasound. Once the artery has been individuated, the dilated testicular veins are individually twice clipped and divided. Division of the veins facilitates exposure and preservation of the artery.

Phlebography

At the end of the procedure we verify the complete ligation of all spermatic veins by means of transfemoral phlebography (Fig. 2). In four cases we found a nonligated spermatic vein. The total number of ligated veins varied from one to five. The venographic procedure requires

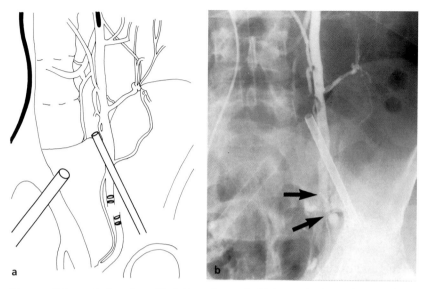

a   b

Fig. 2. a Schematic drawing of b. **b** Transfemoral phlebography is used to verify the complete ligation of all spermatic veins (*arrows*)

15 min. An X-ray check is not always necessary. Venography can be repeated after having clipped the previously nonligated spermatic vein.

Termination of the Procedure

A careful inspection for hemostasis and visceral integrity is performed upon completion of spermatic vein ligation. We prefer to minimize the use of electrocautery to decrease the danger of injuring the spermatic artery. Before inspecting the pelvis the patient is rotated to a neutral position and placed in the reverse Trendelenburg position; any saline or blood that has accumulated during laparoscopy is aspirated. Each instrument port insertion site is then inspected to assess any hemorrhage; for a better view it may be useful to place the laparoscope through the 11-mm midline suprapubic port. We control every trocar extraction directly. Having controlled the scrotum, the CO_2 is removed slowly from the peritoneal cavity. A single fascial no. 1 polyglycolic acid suture is placed at the midline insertion sites that had maintained an access to 11-mm sheaths. The skin is closed with sterile strips or with a subcuticular absorbable suture. A small dressing is applied, and the bladder catheter is removed.

Side Effects

The appearance of carbon dioxide pneumoscrotum has been reported by several authors and is due to the fact that CO_2 may dissect through the internal ring and into the scrotum. Since this causes no significant problems, it cannot be considered a complication. In the presence of pneumoscrotum it is sufficient to squeeze the scrotum before removal of the sheaths to compress the CO_2 back into the peritoneal cavity.

Postoperative Management

Two doses of parenteral antibiotics are administered postoperatively. All patients have tolerated clear fluids on the evening of the procedure and of ambulating. Oral analgesics have been required only in one patient to ease the CO_2 diaphragmatic irritation. A prospective study has compared the preoperative and postoperative values of hematocrit. All patients should undergo repeated blood analyses on the morning after intervention.

Results

Since July 1991 we have performed more than 50 laparoscopic procedures. We followed up 22 patients who had had the same procedures (preoperative abdominal echographic check, Doppler flowmetry of the artery, intraoperative phlebography).

The 6-month follow-up showed resolution of the varicocele in all but one patient, with the disappearance of pain in the patient treated also for this symptom. Three months after intervention one patient showed a recurrence of left varicocele at physical examination; Doppler flowmetry confirmed the presence of a renospermatic reflux. The patient underwent percutaneous spermatic phlebography that revealed the presence of a collateral vein that had not been ligated during laparoscopy. Sclerotherapy allowed the complete occlusion of the vein on an outpatient basis and under local anesthesia. Few changes in testicular size have been noted by means of scrotal ultrasound. In seven cases a compensatory growth was observed; however, in three cases a further atrophy was noted (one of which was the case of persistence of renospermatic reflux, and the other two patients were older than 30). Total operative time ranged from 90 to 150 min. There has been minimal morbidity associated with this procedure. Hypercapnia or respiratory depression has not been encountered. One patient complained of transient shoulder pain and required an oral analgesic. In one case a fall in hematocrit value was evident on the morning after intervention; this patient had complained of abdominal discomfort during the evening and night. No medical therapy was necessary to treat the pain and the transitory anemia.

We repeated Doppler flowmetry of the spermatic arteries in all cases. The procedure was performed by the same operator with the same instrument, and arteries pulses were studied at the same level pre- and postoperatively. In no case did we encounter any changes between the two testes. Patient weight (average 75.1, range 63–98 kg) did not preclude laparoscopic varix ligation. Two patients had undergone previous appendectomy and inguinal surgical ligature. All the men were discharged after 2 days and were able to return to work or school within 5 days.

Discussion

The frequent relationship between varicocele and infertility [9–13] confronts the surgeon with the problem of correcting the varicocele without provoking further damage to fertility.

Varicocele is commonly due to the incompetence or absence of the testicular vein valves [14] and/or to increased hydrostatic pressure [14, 16]. In these cases retroperitoneal spermatic vein ligation [17] may be sufficient if all veins are individuated and ligated. The laparoscopic technique yields the same results as the Palomo approach since both procedures are directed at the spermatic veins proximally to the internal ring. It may offer a number of advantages because it is microscopic and allows the accurate identification of veins, arteries, and lymphatics. However, we prefer sclerotherapy in cases of monolateral left varicocele because of the potential complications of laparoscopy and anesthesia. In Italy there is no need for specialized radiological support, and in our 3000 procedures the failure rate due to technical problems has been very low. We do not consider inadvertent venous perforation as a failure if spermatic reflux is completely abolished. Furthermore, we have learned to avoid misinterpretation of venography due to the frequent proximal location of the valves in the spermatic vein [18]. In addition, we never use any occlusive device and therefore avoid the risk of migration.

In our experience the prevalence of bilateral varicocele is higher than that reported by Dubin and Amelar [19] (14%) and Okuyama et al. [20] (16.6%). Physicians who use diagnostic techniques (e.g., Doppler flowmetry, scrotal ultrasound) other than physical examination surely discover a great number of bilateral varicoceles [7]. Furthermore, the high percentage of bilateral varicocele may explain the pathophysiological mechanism by which bilateral testicular dysfunction, which was formerly considered a unilateral anatomical abnormality, may be produced. We have experienced the difficulty correcting bilateral varicoceles percutaneously, and we now think that laparoscopy can become the gold standard procedure. For this we must be able to: (a) individuate the extrafunicular varicocele preoperatively, (b) identify the artery, (c) prevent the large number of recurrences reported with similar surgical techniques, and (d) minimize the risks associated with laparoscopy.

How To Individuate Extrafunicular Varicocele Preoperatively

Dennison and Tibbs [21] documented the presence of circuitous flow, retrograde down the testicular and anterograde to the cremasteric, pudendal, and finally the iliac vein systems. In such cases ligation of internal spermatic veins is sufficient and does not compromise the normal venous run-off from the testicle. On the other hand, especially in the presence of varicocele and varix at the level of the legs, one must suspect an iliac stasis and a probable extrafunicular varicocele. In these cases the patient must be carefully examined by Doppler flowmetry. If it is not possible to abolish the reflux by strong compression at the level of the internal ring, one should suspect an extrafunicular varicocele. In these cases we prefer to operate at the level of the inguinal channel and have often found dilated extrafunicular veins in the lower part of the inguinal channel that cannot be seen by usual laparoscopic inspection.

How To Identify the Spermatic Arteries During Laparoscopy

Numerous techniques are taught for identifying the spermatic arteries. These methods seek: (a) to avoid prolonged manipulation of the cord, (b) to irrigate the cord with papaverine or lidocaine to diminish vasospasm, (c) to use an intraoperative Doppler (if disposable), (d) to divide the veins up to facilitate exposure and preservation of the arteries. In addition to these procedures, we consider it useful to perform Doppler flowmetry before and after the intervention ensure that no arteries have been damaged.

How To Prevent the Large Number
of Recurrences After High Ligation of Spermatic Veins

Murray et al. [4] studied venographies of 44 recurrent varicoceles in 37 patients and identified three types of patterns: parallel, renal vein, and transscrotal collateral pathways. It is well known that a common cause of failure of the operation is the feeding collateral renospermatic, lumbar, and capsular veins into the internal spermatic vein just proximal to the internal ring [5, 9, 15]. The possible occurrence of left-to-right crossing veins [12] can be well identified and ligated by laparoscopic techniques. The presence of a single vein is clearly less frequent than that of multiple veins. Although the magnification given by laparoscopy allows us better to identify all the veins, we have encountered four cases in which intraoperative phlebography has shown the presence of other collateral veins to be ligated. If the intervention is performed well, intraoperative transfemoral phlebography must not show any presence of veins toward the kidney. To perform left renospermatic phlebography all veins must be interrupted by clips and evidence of collateral veins excluded. In the transfemoral approach one must consider that selective catheterization of the right spermatic vein is mandatory.

How To Minimize the Risks Associated with Laparoscopy

Contributions have been made by numerous authors regarding means by which the risks associated with laparoscopy may be minimized. We think that especially in treating pathologies such as varicocele one must pay particular attention to avoiding complications. For this reason we prefer deep physical examination by means of abdominal ultrasound for ruling out the presence of sometimes nonpalpable pathologies, such as aortic aneurysms, urachal cysts, and solid masses.

Conclusions

The microscopic nature of laparoscopic surgery can enhance the anatomical advantages of this technique (which is essentially a high ligation with decreased morbidity) to improve control of all spermatic veins. Laparoscopy is simple and effective and entails minimal morbidity, but in cases of monolateral left varicocele its cost/benefit ratio is not yet as favorable as that of sclerotherapy. Preoperative abdominal ultrasound, intraoperative phlebography, and Doppler flowmetry can improve the laparoscopic treatment of varicocele. The time invested in any safer procedure is well spent, especially when treating infertile patients with varicocele.

References

1. Winfield HN, Donovan JF, See WA, Loening SA, Williams RD (1991) Urological laparoscopic surgery. J Urol 146:941
2. Hargood PG, Mehan DJ, Worischeck JH, Andrus CH, Parra RO (1992) Laparoscopic varicocelectomy: preliminary report of a new technique. J Urol 147:73–76
3. Donovan JF, Winfield HN (1992) Laparoscopic varix ligation. J Urol 147:77–81
4. Murray RR Jr, Mitchell SE, Radir S, Raufman SL, Chang R, Rinnison ML, Smyth W, White RI Jr (1986) Comparison of recurrent varicocele anatomy following surgery and percutaneous balloon occlusion. J Urol 135:286
5. Raufman SL, Radir S, Barth RH, Smyth JW, Walsh PC, White RI Jr (1983) Mechanisms of recurrent varicocele after balloon occlusion or surgical ligation of the internal spermatic vein. Radiology 147:435
6. Belgrano E, Puppo P, Quattrini S, Trombetta C, Giuliani L (1984) The role of venography and sclerotherapy in the management of varicocele. Eur Urol 10:24
7. McClure RD, Hricak H (1986) Scrotal ultrasound in the infertile man: detection of subclinical unilateral and bilateral varicocele. J Urol 135:711
8. Belgrano E, Puppo P, Quattrini S, Trombetta C, Pittaluga P (1984(19 Microsurgical spermatico-epigastric anastomosis for treatment of varicocele. Microsurgery 5:44
9. Narayan P, Amplatz R, Gonzales R (1991) Varicocele and male subfertility. Fertil Steril 36:92
10. Pryor JL, Howards SS (1988) Varicocele. In: Tanagho EA, Lue TF, McClure RD (eds) Contemporary management of impotence and infertility. Williams and Wilkins, Baltimore, pp. 247–264
11. Hendry WF, Soerville IF, Hall RR, Pugh RCB (1975) Investigation and treatment of the subfertile male. Br J Urol 45:684
12. Cockett ATR, Urry RL, Dougherty RA (1979) The varicocele and semen characteristics. J Urol 121:435
13. Lipshultz LI, Howards SS (1983) Surgical treatment of male infertility. In: Lipschultz LI, Howards SS (eds) Infertility in the male. Churchill Livingstone, New York, pp 343–366
14. Ahlberg NE, Bartley O, Chidekel N (1966) Right and left gonadal veins. An anatomical and statistical study. Acta Radiol 4:593
15. Coolsaet BLRA (1980) The varicocele syndrome: venography determining the optimal level for surgical management. J Urol 124:833
16. Sayfan J, Halevy A, Oland J, Nathan H (1984) Varicocele and left renal vein compression. Fertil Steril 41:411
17. Palomo A (1949) Radical cure of varicocele by a new technique: preliminary report. J Urol 61:604
18. Nadel SN, Hutchins GM, Albertsen PC, White RI Jr (1984) Valves of the internal spermatic vein: potential for misdiagnosis of varicocele by venography. Fertil Steril 41:479
19. Dubin L, Amelar RD (1975) Varicocelectomy as therapy in male infertility: a study of 504 cases. Fertil Steril 26:217

20. Okuyama A, Nakamura M, Namiki M, Takeyama M, Utsunomiya N, Fujioka H, Itatani H, Matsuda M, Matsumoto R, Sonoda T (1988) Surgical repair of varicocele at puberty: preventive treatment for fertility improvement. J Urol 139:562–64

21. Dennison AR, Tibbs DJ (1986) Varicocele and varicose veins compared. A basis for logical surgery. Urology 28:211

Microsurgical Spermatic-Epigastric Anastomosis for Treatment of Varicocele

E. Belgrano, C. Trombetta, S. Siracusano, and G. Savoca

Introduction

The microsurgical anastomosis between the internal spermatic vein and the inferior epigastric vein was first described in the technique of testis autotransplantation. In this surgery, performed in children, the anastomosis is difficult because of the extremely tiny wall of the internal spermatic vein. Straffon and coworkers [11] have therefore maintained that venous drainage via the internal spermatic vein is not strictly necessary for the testis. Occlusion of the internal spermatic vein is commonly performed for varicocele correction, leaving the testis without its major venous pathway. However, Silber's reports [9, 10] and our experimental studies [2] have demonstrated that a certain damage to the autotransplanted testis is always present when the venous anastomosis is not accomplished, and now there is general agreement that the venous drainage of the testis should be restored to normal in testis autotransplantation [4, 10].

Then, why not in varicocele surgery? These new concepts concerning the need for restoration of a good venous drainage after spermatic vein ligation have been developing in recent years and have led to the introduction of new microsurgical techniques at the shunts between one or two veins of the spermatic cord and the saphenous vein [6]. On the basis of our clinical and experimental experience on testis autotransplantation [2–4] we believe that the epigastric vein is the most suitable for the anastomosis with the internal spermatic vein, and therefore we propose the use of this surgical solution also in varicocele surgery.

Microsurgical Technique

Through a standard inguinal incision the external oblique fascia is opened, and the cord structures are mobilized, care being taken to preserve the ilioinguinal nerve. The inferior epigastric vessels are identified and carefully isolated for a length of 3–4 cm. The operating microscope is then introduced into the operating field and under 6–10-fold magnification the spermatic vein(s) are separated from the spermatic artery. In a similar fashion the epigastric vein(s) are separated from the epigastric artery. The internal spermatic vein is divided, and the distal stump, that is, the one further from the testis, is ligated. The epigastric vein is also divided, and the proximal stump that is, the one further from the iliac vein, is ligated. The proximal stump of the spermatic vein is end-to-end anastomosed to the distal stump of the epigastric vein with 9/0 nylon separate stitches under 16-fold magnification. The external spermatic veins are left untouched. The whole operation is summarized schematically in Fig. 1. In the case of multiple spermatic or epigastric veins, the largest vein is selected for the anastomosis, and the others are divided and ligated.

In some cases renospermatic reflux is not the sole cause of varicocele, but a venous hypertension in the left iliac vein strongly contributes to varicocele by iliacospermatic reflux via the external spermatic veins (Fig. 2). In this case ligation of the internal spermatic vein is mandatory, as is ligation of the external spermatic veins. The venous drainage of the testis should therefore be improved by spermaticoepigastric anastomosis, but the epigastric vein drains into the iliac vein and therefore is not suitable for this purpose. However, the proximal stump of the epigastric vein offers a good solution because this vein normally anastomoses with the superior epigastric and mammarian veins and therefore represents a good collateral circle draining into the large veins of the thorax which works, for example, in Budd-Chiari syndrome (Fig. 3). The end-to-end anastomosis between the proximal stump of the spermatic vein and the proximal stump of the epigastric vein is performed with 9/0 separate stitches under 16-fold magnification. In the case of multiple spermatic or/and epigastric veins the largest vein is selected.

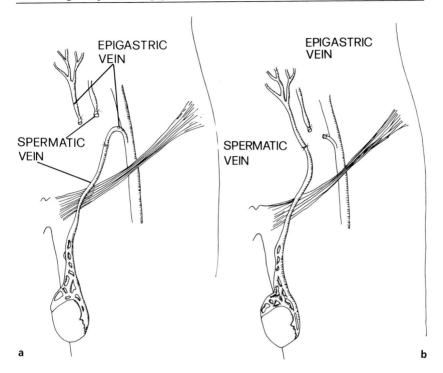

Fig. 1 a,b. Microsurgical spermaticoepigastric anastomosis. **a** The distal stump of the epigastric vein is end-to-end anastomosed with the proximal stump of the spermatic vein. **b** Here the proximal (abdominal) stump of the epigastric vein is used for the anastomosis. This intervention is indicated in type 3 varicocele

Discussion

Several technical considerations demonstrate, in our opinion, that the epigastric vein is the most suitable for anastomosis with the spermatic vein:

- The inguinal approach is advisable in all cases to confirm under direct vision the diagnosis of internal (intrafunicular) or external (extrafunicular) varicocele, and that the epigastric vein lies on the inferior wall of the inguinal channel.
- The epigastric and spermatic veins are so close that any tension of the anastomosis is avoided.

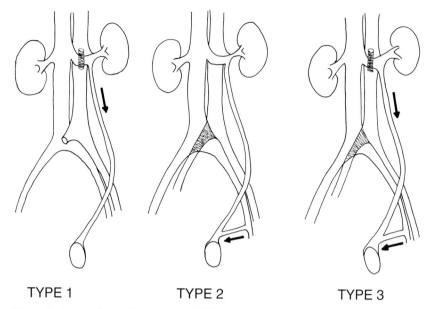

TYPE 1   TYPE 2   TYPE 3

Fig. 2. Pathogenetic mechanisms and different types of varicocele according to the classification of Coolsaet (see text for details)

- The chance to use alternatively the proximal or distal stump of the epigastric vein offers an elegant hemodynamic solution.
- The anastomosis is quite easy because the veins have a similar diameter in the great majority of cases.

The whole operation requires no more than 1 h. The venous flow from the testis is surely enhanced, thus offering better conditions for spermatogenesis. Otherwise, in the case of simple venous ligation, new venous anastomotic connections are established between testis venous circulation and general venous circulation, but this process takes time and cannot be as physiological.

The indications of this technique must be discussed in terms of the pathogenetic mechanism of varicocele. Several venographic studies [1,3,8,13] have demonstrated that there are at least two mechanisms and three distinct types of varicocele.

Fig. 3. Schema of the venous circulation of the abdominal wall. Note the full-channel anastomosis between inferior and superior epigastric vein

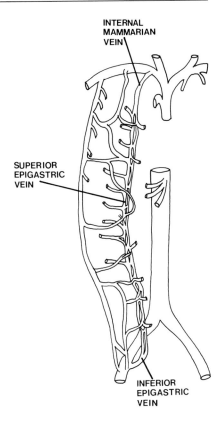

INTERNAL
MAMMARIAN
VEIN

SUPERIOR
EPIGASTRIC
VEIN

INFERIOR
EPIGASTRIC
VEIN

Type 1 Varicocele

The cause of the type 1 varicocele is in the internal spermatic vein itself, with or without an associated proximal nutcracker phenomenon, with compression of the left renal vein at the level of the junction between the aorta and the mesenteric artery and renospermatic reflux [3]. Occlusion of the internal spermatic vein is mandatory, and in many cases this is enough to solve the problem because the venous drainage through the external spermatic veins into the iliac vein is efficient. Occlusion of the internal spermatic vein can be carried out by surgical ligation or by transcatheter sclerotization [5]. Several reports [1,5,12] have demonstrated that sclerotherapy is as efficient as high surgical ligation in removing renospermatic reflux. Therefore it seems perfectly reasonable to perform sclerotherapy in type 1 varicocele whenever a selective and distal catheterization of the internal spermatic vein has been achieved, during the same venographic session. This treatment can be planned on an outpatient basis, and its additional cost with respect to venography is minimal. In cases of technically impossible or unsuccessful sclerotherapy open surgery must be planned.

In our opinion the technique of Ivanissevich [7] should be abandoned because it does not offer the possibility to confirm the venographic diagnosis under direct vision, as is the case by opening the inguinal channel; at best it gives the same result as sclerotherapy. The microsurgical anastomosis between the internal spermatic vein and iliac stump of the epigastric vein represents a real progress with respect to the simple ligation and should be the treatment of choice in cases of type 1 varicocele where it is impossible to carry out sclerotherapy. In other words, varicocele surgery cannot be limited today to occlusion of the pathological circulation because microsurgery offers the possibility to create a new venous drainage to the testis.

Type 2 Varicocele

A very small percentage of varicoceles are due only to a distal (low) nutcracker phenomenon created by the iliac artery which runs anteriorly to it [3]. There is no renospermatic reflux. In these cases the internal spermatic vein should not be ligated, and surgery should be limited to ligation of the external spermatic veins, which are involved by the hypertension in the left iliac vein. However, in many cases the diagnosis of type 2 varicocele is made after an unsuccessful high ligation of the internal spermatic vein. These cases should be treated as type 3 varicoceles.

Type 3 Varicocele

Type 3 variocele is a combination of types 1 and 2 [3]. Sclerotherapy is not sufficient to cure type 3 varicoceles because it does not provide correction of the lower obstruction. The anastomosis between the testicular stump of the internal spermatic vein and the abdominal stump of the inferior epigatric vein offers a good chance of restoring to normal the testis venous drainage. Through the anastomotic connections between the inferior epigastric vein and the superior epigastric vein, and then the mammarian vein, the blood coming from the testis can enter a venous system connected to the superior vena cava, whose pressure is much lower. Valves are present in the epigastric vein, but only in the part close to the iliac vein. These must be sought and carefully avoided. The technical performance of the microsurgical anastomosis entails no particular problem. Care must also be taken in ligating all the external spermatic veins. This new technique thus offers much greater guarantee of success than simple ligation and, in our opinion, should be adopted in all cases of type 3 varicocele.

References

1. Belgrano E, Carmignani G, Puppo P, Quattrini S, Trombetta C (1982) Transcatheter treatment of varicocele. International Congress series no 596. Therapy in andrology. Excerpta Medica, Amsterdam, pp 233–238
2. Carmignani G, Belgrano E, Puppo P, Bentivoglio G (1979) Hoden-auto-transplantation. Eine experimentelle Untersuchung am Hund. Akt Urol 10:321–327
3. Coolsaet BL (1980) The varicocele syndrome: venography determining the optimal level for surgical management. J Urol 124:833–839
4. Giuliani L, Carmignani G, Belgrano E, Puppo P (1981) Autotransplantation des testicules dans la cryptorchidie abdominale. J Urol (Paris) 87:279–281
5. Iaccarino V (1980) A nonsurgical treatment of varicocele: transcatheter sclerotherapy of gonadal veins. Ann Radiol 23:269–370
6. Ishigami K, Yoshida Y, Hirooka M (1970) A new operation for varicocele: use of microvascular anastomosis. Surgery 67:620–630
7. Ivanissevich O (1960) Left varicocele due to reflux. Experience with 4470 operative cases in forty-two years. J Int Coll Surg 34: 742–755
8. Ponthieu A, Huguet JG (1976) Varicocèle gauche et stase veineuse iliaque. J Urol Nephrol 3:187–200
9. Silber SJ, Kelly J (1978) Successful autotransplantation of an intra-abdominal testis to the scrotum by microvascular techniques. J Urol 115: 115–119
10. Silber SJ (1981) The intra-abdominal testes: microvascular autotransplantation. J Urol 125:329–333
11. Wacksman J, Dinner M, Straffon RA (1978) Testicular autotransplant in prune belly disease. Presented at annual meeting of the American Urological Association. Washington DC, May 21–25

12. Zeitler E, Jecht E, Richter EI, Seyferth W (1980) Selective sclerotherapy of the internal spermatic vein in patients with varicoceles. Ann Radiol 23: 371–376
13. Zerhouni EA, Siegelman SS, Walsh PC, White RI (1980) Elevated pressure in the left renal vein in patients with varicocele: preliminary observations. J Urol 123: 512–514

Subject Index

Printing: Saladruck, Berlin
Binding: Buchbinderei Lüderitz & Bauer, Berlin